HOW I CONQUERED
SCHIZOPHRENIA

HOW I CONQUERED
SCHIZOPHRENIA

NANCY STACKHOUSE

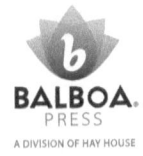

BALBOA.
PRESS
A DIVISION OF HAY HOUSE

Balboa Press books may be ordered through booksellers or by contacting:

Balboa Press
A Division of Hay House
1663 Liberty Drive
Bloomington, IN 47403
www.balboapress.com
1-(877) 407-4847

ISBN: 978-1-4525-6297-1 (e)
ISBN: 978-1-4525-6296-4 (sc)
ISBN: 978-1-4525-6298-8 (hc)

Library of Congress Control Number: 2012921141

Printed in the United States of America

Balboa Press rev. date: 11/14/2012

DEDICATION PAGE

This book is dedicated first to my mother, Helen Duke. You were there for me to provide any help you possibly could during the years I suffered from schizophrenia. I do not think I would have survived without you.

And I dedicate this book to my psychiatrist, Dr. H. Lee Mitchell. You took the time to counsel me and recommend outstanding books for reading in addition to prescribing medications. I so appreciate the extra time you gave to help me fully understand the disease, to regain my self-esteem, and develop what you called "insight into the disorder." You expertly oversaw the "weaning off" of both the antipsychotic and antidepressant medications I was taking.

This book is also dedicated to my brother, Steve Duke, who has passed to the other side. Thank you for continuing to visit and provide me warmth, smiles, compassion, support, and beautiful memories from when you were here on Earth.

Most importantly, this book is dedicated to my husband, Scott Stackhouse. Your unconditional love for those people and places you hold dear has been a true inspiration for me to develop that beautiful characteristic as well. You are the soul mate I searched for and am so blessed to have in my life.

ACKNOWLEDGMENTS

There are many friends and family members I would like to thank for taking the time to read the beginning drafts of this manuscript and provide feedback, suggestions, and wonderful insights for improvement. Jackie Earnhart, especially, was instrumental in helping me believe that my story should be told and could help others. With my permission, she shared one of my initial drafts with friends of her, Maggie and Richard, who have a son in his twenties who suffers from schizophrenia. Maggie and Richard guided me to include portions in the book that would be helpful to family members and caretakers of those with mental illness and to discuss more in-depth the longstanding and continuing stigma attached to the mental illness label of schizophrenia in particular.

Others who provided helpful feedback included colleagues and friends, Toni Rantala, Evie Garcia, Paige Miller-Leister, Dona Lewinger, and Lynne Cockrum-Murphy. My husband, Scott Stackhouse, my mother-in-law, Cherie Stackhouse, my sister-in-law, Kristie Bramley, and my mother, Helen Duke, have all enthusiastically supported the writing of this book. Several people, including my sister, Marla Duke, have expressed their appreciation of the "Reader's Workbook" opportunities included throughout the book.

CONTENTS

INTRODUCTION

This story is a true life, autobiographical account of my experiences, primarily, with the psychological disorder called schizophrenia including the development of the illness, the diagnosis and treatment, and my ultimate complete recovery. A brief thumbnail definition of schizophrenia taken from the National Alliance on Mental Illness website is: "Schizophrenia is a serious mental illness that affects 2.4 million American adults over the age of 18. Psychosis is a common symptom of schizophrenia. Psychosis is defined as the experience of loss of contact with reality and usually involves hallucinations and delusions." The Mayo Clinic website defines schizophrenia as: "A group of severe brain disorders in which people interpret reality abnormally. Schizophrenia may result in some combination of hallucinations, delusions, and disordered thinking and behavior." A more in-depth description and explanation of mental illnesses including both schizophrenia and depression are presented in chapter two.

Of utmost importance in this book are the descriptions of several strategies used by me to become fully free of schizophrenia and the medications used to treat it. The strategies are explained in such a way that the reader might be able to apply these strategies to his or her own life. The primary purpose of this book is to share these sometimes nontraditional strategies with those who suffer from schizophrenia along with their families, friends, and health care practitioners so all of their lives can be more joyous and fulfilling.

There are many books and resources available today that illuminate the disorder of schizophrenia. While my book shares information regarding various symptoms of schizophrenia, its prevalence, and prognoses, it is not a scientific book on the illness. I wish to share my personal experiences with schizophrenia as well as the mental illness of depression only because I have been successful at overcoming both. Because schizophrenia presents itself in many different forms in terms of symptoms and severity, the information I present here may not work for all schizophrenics or those suffering from depression. Through the hard personal work of changing my thinking, changing my behaviors, and opening myself up to being healed, I have been able to release myself of all symptoms of schizophrenia and depression and all medications used to treat them. While I have earned a doctor of education degree, I am not a doctor of medicine. Therefore, a disclaimer is made here to any and all who suffer from mental illness and a strong recommendation is made that professional medical assistance be obtained first and foremost from a licensed medical family practice doctor who may then refer one to a licensed psychiatrist.

Some readers may gain insights into their own thinking and behavior through reading my story, and, thus, be able to make their own progress in overcoming mental illness. I believe each reader will gain something different from my book depending on his or her own experiences with schizophrenia or depression. Still other readers might know of a relative or friend in their lives who might benefit from reading or hearing about my story. And another group of readers may find that they resonate with the unconventional healing methods described herein and/or be interested in learning more about them. In particular, I wish to point out to the reader that, in chapter eight, I detail a process called "The Raven Clan Clearing." This is a healing process that I learned about through a healer I knew who recommended it. It took time for me to learn about the concept and "wrap my mind around" its possibility. I would understand that you, the reader, may or may not resonate with this phenomenon. Therefore, please skip over it if you find it too hard to believe and please take from the book only those ideas that you find helpful.

This book is also offered to those who provide treatment to individuals with schizophrenia or depression. The story I present and the strategies I use might be shared by medical professionals with their patients in order to help them recover as much as possible from these debilitating disorders. I had what could be termed mild cases of both schizophrenia and depression. I was never hospitalized, institutionalized, or unable to work. The information I present is most appropriate for those in similar circumstances. A larger proportion of those suffering from schizophrenia and depression are not as fortunate. They are living the nightmare of institutionalization, unemployment, poverty, homelessness, and prison. My greatest hope is that my story might provide small amounts of relief or even inspiration to these individuals along with a huge amount of compassion and understanding for them. HOPE is the magical word here that is foremost in importance to my message to readers.

I have included in an appendix numerous websites and resources that might be of assistance to those suffering from schizophrenia, depression, or any other mental illness. As I will explain in the book, the first, best, and most important step to recovery is getting help. Websites, resources, and support groups listed in the appendix might prove helpful to families, friends, health care providers, and caretakers as well. Lastly, I have shared in the references and recommended reading section at the end of the book the many sources and materials that I have either cited within this book, read, listened to, or used that have so positively supported my recovery and continued maintenance of positive mental, emotional, spiritual, and physical health.

Thank you from the bottom of my heart for allowing me to share my story.

CHAPTER ONE

Stressful Times

Anyone ever born on this planet has to believe that it is a stressful place to live. While we can all agree that it can be difficult to live on Earth, we can further agree that the stressful conditions in which we find ourselves require response in one form or another. We might even agree that certain responses to stress, indeed, are healthier than other responses. Where all of this agreement breaks down, however, is in the vast array of actual choices we make as individuals coping with the stressful times in our lives. My story of stress is not unique nor is the resulting effect of the stress which included depression, auditory hallucinations, and a diagnosis of schizophrenia. What is fairly unique is my eventual conquering and releasing of these disorders. I believe others with mental illness as well as their families, friends, caretakers, and medical professionals might wish to explore and use some of the strategies explained herein that led to my complete recovery from mental illness. My intention is to give HOPE to anyone and everyone touched by mental illness and that is why this story is told.

EARLY YEARS

My parents were married immediately after graduating from the high school where they met in Dayton, Ohio. With high school educations, my father worked in civil service for the government and my mother worked as a grocery store cashier. We were a middle class family from, primarily,

1

Irish descent. When I was three, my oldest brother was six, my next oldest brother was five, my sister was four, and my youngest brother was just being born. We were very close in age.

My earliest memory of purposefully coping with stress is of sucking my thumb at about age three or four. This seemed to disturb my parents as they attempted several interventions to try and get me to stop. I was the fourth of five children born to young parents in the mid-fifties and I was the only one who sucked my thumb. Throughout my childhood, I was repeatedly called the "sensitive one" by most everyone in my family. I remember a time when all of the children were given the task of pulling weeds from our yard. Within a short time, my eyes swelled shut. My parents took me to the doctor who explained that I had contracted poison ivy from the air. After shots and medicine, it went away, and my parents, thankfully, didn't require me to pull weeds anymore. I did continue to get poison ivy whenever I was near it, but I was better able to prevent serious outbreaks by taking a poison ivy extract prescribed by one doctor my mother took me to. There was another time when I started breaking out all over when my mother changed our bath soap. Again, the doctor said I was allergic, so my mother had to find a new soap that I was not allergic to.

But, what I remember being most sensitive to was my parents' continual arguing and fighting, and I think I did not deal with the stress of this very well. The arguing and fighting were, from what I could understand, basically, due to my father's drinking. My father has suffered from alcoholism all of his adult life. His father was an alcoholic as well. While many children of alcoholics learn to cope with the stresses of life by becoming alcoholics themselves, a choice I made early on was not to drink alcohol. I especially didn't like the smell of stale beer.

When I was six, my father brought home a huge upright piano that he bought from someone's basement sale for ten dollars. He and my mother encouraged my older brothers and sister to play and take lessons, but none of them was really interested. I remember being very interested in playing the piano and my parents signed me up for lessons at the local church which I enjoyed tremendously. Throughout this chapter, I will identify ten wonderful gifts in my life that have influenced me positively in the ways I have learned to handle stress. This piano was gift number one. Playing piano has been a huge gift to me in my life for many reasons. I have feelings of joy whenever I play. I also feel creative as I play piano. My self-confidence has been enhanced because many have appreciated and applauded my ability including my father. I performed at piano recitals and played in my grade school and high school orchestras. I developed an interest, again, at an early age, in listening to classical music which has been very relaxing for me. Later in life, when I was a schoolteacher, I provided piano accompaniment for our high school jazz ensemble. I continue to enjoy playing jazz piano and listening to jazz as well as many other genres of music. I believe that playing a musical instrument and enjoying all types of music allow one to socialize more easily. This simple interest at an early age in playing piano proved to be a healthy strategy for stress relief throughout my lifetime. I remember when I was older, graduated from college, working as a schoolteacher, and living in my first apartment in Phoenix, Arizona, the first piece of furniture I purchased was a piano that took me two years of monthly payments to buy.

When I was nine, my family moved to a larger house in Dayton, Ohio. The arguing and fighting between my parents continued and seemed to be constant. There seemed to always be a sense of tension and darkness in the house. Later in life, my friend, Mary Ann, who had lived across the street from our house when we were young commented that our house always appeared very dark inside. I remember going over to Mary Ann's house frequently because I felt more joy and safety there.

Each of my siblings dealt with the continual arguing and fighting between my parents differently. It seemed to me that all three of my brothers were able to ignore the fighting and retreated to their bedroom to sleep or listen to music. My sister and I seemed to be most affected. We might be kept up all night listening to the fighting. Sometimes, my sister and I would take turns making up stories of being sick to go out and tell our parents so they would focus on us instead of fighting with each other. This strategy worked a few times, but soon proved to be no longer effective. I remember many nights when our mother would drive her car a few streets over from where we lived so she could get a little sleep before needing to get up for work the next morning. My sister and I would sometimes wrap ourselves up in blankets and walk around the neighborhood looking for her car. We usually found her and offered her sympathy and support.

When my sister, Marla, was twelve, she and my mother registered at the local YMCA to take a yoga class. My mother wanted to register them both in an exercise class and yoga was the only one available. After one session, my mother decided that she really didn't like yoga, and allowed me to take her place for the rest of the classes along with my sister. This turned out to be the second gift in my life that has helped me handle stress.

For anyone who has not taken a basic hatha yoga class, usual activities include deep breathing, stretches, postures, balances, and poses. The class usually concludes with students lying on their backs on their mats with their eyes closed and the teacher talking them through a guided visualization or deep relaxation. Looking back, I realize that it was, basically, a meditation. The first time I experienced this, at age eleven, I remember being in such a profound state of peace and I thought to myself, "Wow! This is home! This is a place I can go to at any time when things get too stressful and crazy in my family." I have either practiced or taught hatha yoga nearly every day of my life since age eleven. In many ways, I believe it has literally saved my life. Another reason why yoga has been so beneficial to me throughout my lifetime is that it has allowed me to meet so many peaceful and health-minded people, again, allowing me to socialize, feel happier, and remain more connected to my community. I always feel happy when I'm doing yoga.

Also, at about this age, I began to really get into walking whenever possible to escape the negative energies in the house. I would volunteer to walk down to the mailbox or to the grocery store just to get away from the fighting. One Saturday afternoon, as I was walking home from the store, I could hear my parents screaming and fighting halfway down the street. I remember thinking to myself that I had been born into the wrong family, and I told myself, "When I grow up and move out, I will never live like this. I will never live in a house where there is all this yelling, screaming, and fighting."

Now I do not want to give the impression that everything was always terrible during my childhood. I believe my parents did the best they could under the circumstances. They encouraged all of us to do well in school and earn good grades. They taught us responsibility in working around the house and we were expected to complete regular chores. We went to major league baseball games and on summer vacations. We had good Christmases and holidays and regularly saw our grandparents, aunts, uncles, and cousins.

In particular, I remember spending time at my grandmother's house (on my mother's side). I loved her so much. I always felt relaxed there. I remember taking naps as a child in her spare bedroom where she kept her now antique Singer sewing machine. I felt peaceful just looking around the room and out the windows. She would let me bake and cook with her and she was so patient. She had only a third-grade education, but she was the wisest person I have ever known and I consider her the third gift in my life for being such a wonderful role model. She also provided me with unconditional love. I never had to do anything to earn her love. Everyone, child or adult, needs people in their lives who offer unconditional love. Having these wonderful people in our lives then allows us the capacity to learn to give unconditional love to others. Even though she is no longer living, I still feel her love, nurturing support, and encouragement around me. Many times in my life, when things get stressful, I need only think of her to feel better.

At about age thirteen, in addition to continually being accused of being "too sensitive" by immediate members of my family, I also remember being told that I was "too smart for my own good." I had always achieved extremely well in school. I actually loved school. It was a place to get away from the craziness of my home life. Enjoying school so much probably played a big part in influencing me to become a school teacher. It was during this time that I began to internalize the stress from home and allow it to make me sick. I developed daily stomach aches and was diagnosed with a peptic ulcer which I suffered from until I moved away to college at age eighteen.

In high school, I was fortunate to be placed in honors English and math classes. There, I was challenged to work and think very hard and I was encouraged by thoughtful and insightful teachers to live up to my intellectual potential. I believe my relatively high intelligence is the fourth gift in life that has contributed greatly to my ability to handle stress. My intelligence, indeed, has led to feelings of success and accomplishment throughout my life, especially with regard to my education and career. I believe my logic and intelligence have helped me choose differently than many of my family members and to make positive decisions about those with whom I choose to have relationships (although I have definitely made some poor decisions). All of my siblings and I were involved in high school activities. The brother I was closest to, Steve, played football, wrestled, and was class president. My sister, Marla, and I were cheerleaders. I wrote for the school newspaper and served as student council president. I think it was beneficial for all of the children to be so involved and productive in school.

During high school, friends would regularly invite us to spend the night or have a sleepover at their houses. But, it was very difficult to return the invitations. We could not dare ask a friend to spend the night at our house for fear that our father would come home drunk, fight with our mother, and then nearly burn the house down with his late night cooking because he would fall asleep with the stove unwatched. I would attend school almost every day smelling like smoke – either from cigarettes because both of my parents smoked or from stove fires.

Even though my father was an alcoholic, he managed to be successful in holding his civil service job with the government. While a good portion of his earnings was earmarked for alcohol, cigarettes, membership in the Eagles club, golfing, and bowling, he was actually quite good with money. He contributed heavily to his credit union, has never been in debt, paid cash for everything, and, to my knowledge, has never owned a credit card. He was a high school graduate, a gifted artist and gymnast, and attended several college classes. He always wanted his five children to do well in school and offered to pay four years of college tuition for each of us. My mother was expected to pay half. She was still working full time in the grocery business and earned a good salary. If we wanted to attend a university away from home, we needed to save money from summer work and part time jobs to pay for room, board, and books.

My oldest brother, Frankie, attended a couple of freshman level college classes, but dropped out. He has spent most of his adult life working in grocery stores, hospitals, and driving school buses and I have not had contact with him in person, by telephone, or by mail since about 1991. My second oldest brother, Steve, was recruited to wrestle for a university ninety miles north of our hometown. Steve was very successful as a wrestler. I enjoyed watching him compete. He was not as successful academically, however, and dropped out of college in his sophomore year. He spent most of his adult life running his own small businesses in office cleaning and home nursing. For the most part, he was very successful and happy running his businesses. He cared a great deal for his employees and clients. My older sister, Marla, attended one year of art school before marrying her high school sweetheart and joining the Army with him. After two children, she attended college part time until she earned her bachelor's degree in art education. Marla has spent most of her adult life working very successfully as either a teacher or administrator for a federally funded education program for disadvantaged preschoolers. I was able to take full advantage of my parents' offer to pay my college tuition for four years. I very much appreciated the sacrifices they made to do this for me.

OFF TO COLLEGE

The day I went off to college was one of the happiest days of my life. I could not wait to be on my own. I felt such a sense of freedom. I began studying pre-law, primarily, because my father wanted me to become a lawyer. I guess I really knew since I was about ten or eleven years of age that I wanted to be a teacher. I used to make up worksheets and "play school" with the younger children across the street and grade their papers. By my junior year in college, it was necessary for me to declare my major. Even though my father was worried that I would not earn adequate money as a teacher, he agreed that I could become one.

My junior and senior years of college were fun, exciting, and memorable, and, also, a time during which I experienced great spiritual growth. Even though I was working several part time jobs on campus to help fund my room, board, and books, I maintained a fairly balanced life between studying, working, dating, and cheerleading. I would also regularly visit the music building to play piano in one of the practice rooms. I even performed in public at a university "Open Mike" night. I taught hatha yoga classes on campus and met interesting students and professors who attended my classes.

During all of my years in college, I maintained a close relationship with my second oldest brother, Steve. He and I played chess together as children. We looked a lot alike and, when we were younger, people would sometimes ask if we were twins. As we got older, he and I would attend many "spiritual" type activities. We would sometimes meditate together in the same room and also long distance to connect telepathically. We would go to the local yoga ashram for chanting and vegetarian food. My brother read many esoteric and spiritual books and would share the information with me. In particular, I remember he read books by Carlos Castaneda and Ram Dass. My brother also became a Bahai which is a follower of the teachings of Baha'u'llah, a Persian who lived in the mid-1800's. During my junior year of college, I became a Bahai as well and my brother and I made several trips to Wilmette, Illinois, to visit the Bahai Temple.

It was during this time that I began to regularly meditate nearly every day. I view my brother, Steve, with all of the love and opportunities he opened up to me, as the fifth great gift in my life and learning to meditate through him as the sixth gift. Even though he was not able to finish college, he was extremely supportive of my doing so. In our dysfunctional, alcoholic family, Steve was the jokester, the one who made everyone laugh and cheered everyone up. He was one of the most generous people I have ever known and I feel blessed to have had him in my life. Later in this book, I will talk about his suicide at the age of 48 and how it affected my life. I would also like to mention here that, although I believe I grew up in a dysfunctional family, I have always loved my mother and father very much. I know they did the best they could. They, themselves, grew up in dysfunctional families and had little guidance or opportunity to learn how to create a thriving and functional family.

Between my junior and senior years in college in Ohio, I had the opportunity to visit my aunt and cousins in Scottsdale, Arizona (where I now live). My Aunt Juanita had lost my uncle to a heart attack earlier that spring and was devastated with having to deal with his death and the aftermath of sorting out finances, land deals, etc. I was having difficulty securing a summer job with the government for which I had worked the previous two summers (at a defense facility and an Air Force base). We were in a severe recession in the late seventies in the Midwest and across the country and it proved incredibly difficult for anyone to find a job. I still had my part time work at college beginning in the fall. So, I decided to take advantage of a summer nationwide special offer to take a Greyhound bus for $50 to anywhere in the continental United States. I chose Scottsdale, Arizona, to see if I could help my aunt and cousins in any way and also to possibly obtain a summer job there.

As the bus drove into Phoenix, Arizona, I arrived with severely swollen ankles from the twenty-eight hour bus ride. I also remember coming to the realization that I did not know that the sun could shine until coming to the Southwest. In the Midwest, it always seemed to be overcast, rainy, and gloomy. I loved Arizona from the beginning – all the mountains, the blue skies, and the wide open spaces. I knew I had to move there after college to become a teacher.

I was only in Scottsdale for about three weeks that summer. I tried to help my aunt (who was my mother's older sister) as much as I could. I even worked as a waitress for eleven days at a local restaurant (being a waitress was very hard work and I definitely appreciate those able to do it for a living). But, the government called with news of a summer position for me back home if I was interested. I was able to fly back (it was my first plane ride at age 21). My Aunt Juanita sent me applications to teach in school districts in Arizona (especially the Phoenix area) and I spent my senior year of college making plans to move west after graduation. I think of my aunt as the seventh wonderful gift in my life and thank her for being the one responsible for my attraction and subsequent move to Arizona. The mountains, atmosphere, and sunsets have given me immeasurable stress relief throughout my adult life. My aunt also provided me with unconditional support and love. She was fun to go shopping with, had a great sense of humor, had a heart of gold, and was a joy to be around.

MOVING WEST

The day of my college graduation from Ohio Northern University, my oldest brother, Frankie, and my mother, Helen, informed me that my mother was going to move west with me. I will be honest and say that I really did not want her to come. But, she had been in a miserable marriage with my father for 26 years and she decided to leave him and get a divorce. Since my Aunt Juanita in Scottsdale, Arizona, was my mother's sister, my mother thought it would be good to stay with my aunt until my mother secured a new job and could live on her own. My father knew that I was moving west, but he had no idea that my mother was coming with me. She waited until he left for work, we loaded up the car, and we began our three day drive west. Mother cried the entire way and for the first year we lived in the Arizona. I tried to help and support her as much as I could as did my aunt. It was a very tough time for my mom.

We stayed with my Aunt Juanita and cousins for approximately four months. I obtained a job as a receptionist for a vitamin company two days after we arrived in Scottsdale on May 25, 1978. My mom secured a job addressing envelopes and was able to work from home. I applied for several full time elementary teaching positions in the Phoenix area, but, the country was in a deep recession during this time and teaching jobs were very hard to come by.

One very hot August day in 1978, I was reading the newspaper want ads and rental columns and was intuitively led to notice an advertisement for a mobile home rental available in south Scottsdale. Mom and I made an appointment and took a tour of the home. We decided to move in and did so in early September, 1978. For a while, we had a little trouble making ends meet with our modest incomes. I decided to write a letter to my father and asked him if he could send a check for $200 each month to my mother as a sort of "alimony" payment until their divorce was final. Dad did so without hesitation. He also came to visit me once in the fall of 1979 right after I landed my first teaching position.

My first full time teaching position in Arizona was as a sixth-grade teacher at a school district in the Phoenix area. I loved teaching. During my second year, I began taking a graduate level education course at Arizona State University where I met my first boyfriend in Arizona. He was a teacher, too, and the gift he gave to me was in introducing me to hiking, mountain climbing, and camping. We only dated for about a year and our breakup was very painful for me. I was madly in love with him, but he thought I was too "spiritual" for him. Looking back, I know that a long term relationship with him would never have worked because he did not view females as equals as he was rather chauvinistic and we did not agree on much of anything.

I remember, in particular, a time in late May, 1980, just as the school year was ending, my boyfriend shared with me that he was planning to be away for much of the summer hiking the Grand Tetons in Wyoming, Mt. Whitney in California, and various other hikes out of state, thus, making him unavailable to see me very much, if at all, over the summer. I responded that I was disappointed, but understood his love of hiking. The next day, I received my monthly *Bahai Newsletter* where I discovered an opportunity to teach summer classes at a Bahai school called Green Acre in Eliot, Maine. I interviewed over the telephone and was offered the job for the summer. I was not scheduled to begin my second year of teaching full time as a sixth grade teacher until late August, so the summer job offer was perfect!

I was so excited to get to travel to Maine for the summer! But, when I shared this wonderful news with my boyfriend, his response was, "Oh, no, you are not. I did not say you could go." I explained that, since he was planning to be away hiking for most of the summer, I would, indeed, be going to Maine for the summer. My boyfriend did not like this news and broke up with me. I went to Maine and had a wonderful time. I even dated a few Bahai fellows that I met and worked with there. After I was in Maine for about four weeks, my Phoenix boyfriend called me numerous times and told me how much he loved and missed me and wanted to get back together. I really loved and missed him, too, and agreed to try again. When I returned home to Phoenix later that summer, I felt a "spiritual high" from my great time at the Bahai summer school and on the Maine coast. After a few more dates, my boyfriend declared that I had become, as I mentioned earlier, "too spiritual," so we broke up permanently. However, I am thankful to him for introducing me to the great outdoors. I continue to be an avid hiker to this day and enjoy traveling all around the Southwest. I think all people benefit from getting outdoors, seeing nature, feeling the sunshine, and looking at a beautiful blue sky. It just makes you feel good and feel as though you have been on a little vacation from your stress. Hiking, mountain climbing, or any kind of outdoor or indoor exercise improves your health and brightens your spirits. Almost every person in my family has had to struggle with being overweight for much of their lives. I am nearly the only one who has maintained a normal weight and I attribute that success to daily exercise and eating healthy (most of the time). I believe a major source of depression for children and adults is being overweight and any efforts one can make to exercise daily and monitor his or her calorie consumption can only contribute to a healthier, happier, and more balanced life.

It was at about this time that I became interested in special education and started a master's degree program at Arizona State University in this field. To help pay for my tuition, I worked part time at a local hospital in the laboratory admitting outpatients for lab work on the weekends. This is a time during which I started feeling out of balance in my life. I was teaching fulltime, attending graduate school in the evenings, and working at the hospital part time on the weekends. I had little, if any, time left over for fun, friends, or exercise. I began taking pain relievers that had caffeine as an ingredient to help me stay awake. I have never been a coffee or tea drinker so I obtained my caffeine through pain relievers.

During my fifth year of teaching, I completed my master's degree in special education from Arizona State University and was given a special education teaching position by my school district. I taught learning disabled and emotionally handicapped children in kindergarten through grade three. During this time, I met someone who I then thought was the "love of my life." I will not go into all of the details, but the relationship ended badly and I believe it was at this time that I experienced a minor emotional breakdown. I was so devastated. I began to believe that I would never love again, and, worse yet, believed that I could never be loved. This huge loss of self-esteem paved the way for the mental illness that followed in my life some twelve years later.

I tried to pick myself back up by throwing myself into teaching. I had worked for one school district for six years. However, a professor friend of mine and a previous principal who had moved to a different school district in the Phoenix area both encouraged me to apply to this particular district. The pay was better and the district had an excellent reputation. I applied, was hired, and worked for this second school district for fourteen years.

GOING INTO ISOLATION

I began work at my new job as a special education teacher in 1985. I enjoyed the work, the children, the other teachers, but, I felt sort of empty in my personal life. I still had a low self-esteem when it came to feeling successful in personal relationships. Where I always found a great amount of success, however, was in my education. Earning a higher degree was also a way of earning more money in my school district. So, I began my doctoral program at Northern Arizona University in the area of curriculum and instruction. I took courses part time for several years.

During this time, I developed a great friendship with a fellow teacher at my school named Mary. Our teaching philosophies were similar and she was instrumental in getting me to "go out and play" more in life. We went on several hiking trips and ski trips which were great fun. I was a bridesmaid in her wedding and we have remained close, supportive friends all of these years. She was the matron of honor in my wedding in 2009. I consider her the ninth wonderful gift in my life. She is dependable, honest, positive, and supportive and I greatly appreciate her. It makes a huge difference in my life to know that, if I ever get really down and discouraged, I call her and receive unconditional love and support as well as on target advice.

In the early 1990's, I completed my doctoral comprehensive exams and was well into the work of my dissertation. I was still teaching fulltime although I had returned to regular education and was teaching second grade. Completing the dissertation was a huge amount of work. I would teach all week and then go up to my family's cabin north of the city every weekend to research and write. The cabin is pretty remote and one can tend to feel isolated if visiting alone. I think at this time I may have isolated myself too much. I was becoming too much of an "academic" and neglecting my emotions as well as my spirit. I seemed to purposely avoid coming into contact with people. I dated little or not at all. I cannot stress enough how hard it was on me to complete and finish my dissertation and doctorate. My dissertation ended up being over 500 pages long. I worked on it for over three years while teaching fulltime. I would highly recommend to anyone who is working fulltime and going to school for any degree be sure to take time to exercise, eat healthfully, spend some time with family and friends, strengthen your spirit in whatever way is best for you, have some fun, and try to establish some sort of balance in your life.

After completing my doctorate in 1995, I continued working as a teacher, however, I began pursuing teaching positions at the university level. After several failed attempts, this was the point at which I think I began to go into a depression. I was not happy as a school teacher anymore (it seemed to me that I had a larger proportion of problem students in my classroom than other teachers did because I had a background in special education and was a good disciplinarian), I was unmarried and about to turn 40, and I was also carrying a certain amount of debt due to overspending and paying for my doctoral tuition and work. Although I did not realize it at the time, I think this was when I began having auditory hallucinations. I lived in a condominium that I owned and often thought that my neighbors were fighting and yelling. Sometimes I would have family members come over to see if they could hear anything and they never could.

BREAKING FROM REALITY

In 1998, during my nineteenth year as a successful school teacher, I had my break from reality and development of mental illness. I had continued my pursuit of a university teaching position, and had been invited as a finalist for on-campus interviews at a small university in Georgia. I was very disappointed when I was not chosen. I was at a very low point when the school year ended in May, 1998.

In June, the auditory hallucinations descended upon me full force. Looking back, it was fortunate that I was not working due to summer vacation. Every night at my condominium I thought I was hearing fighting from neighbors upstairs. I would confront my neighbors and they would deny my accusations. When the fighting was so bad that I could not sleep, I decided to go and spend time at the family cabin where I thought it would be peaceful. At the cabin, I again would hear fighting from what I thought were the people in the cabin next door. I would think that they were fighting inside their cabin, outside their cabin, up on the road, and in their car. But, their lights were not on and there were no cars around. I would imagine that they were hiding their car and keeping their lights off. I would think they were talking about me and planning to come over to kill me with a gun. I imagined they were spying on me with secret cameras. I was into full paranoia. At one point, I even called 911 because I knew they were going to kill me. The sheriff and even a helicopter came. They found nothing. The neighbors were actually in another state for the summer. All I could do was cry.

I returned to my condominium where, in my mind, the fighting continued. I called 911 there as well. The police came and could discover nothing. I was desperately sleep deprived. I started spending nights at my mother's house in hopes that I could get some sleep there. She was very worried about me and her concern was a huge gift to me. Although my mother and I have had some differences of opinion over the years, I do know that she loves me and would do just about anything for me if I asked. I know I have been a huge support to her as well.

About two weeks into this paranoia, I started noticing the fighting "voices" as I was driving my car. This was when I realized that something was really wrong. I understood then that the voices were not coming from outside of me, but from within me. This was very scary. The voices also started to focus on me and anything I was doing. They would say derogatory and self-deprecating things. They would tell me how fat I was and, at the time, I weighed 110 pounds. My current weight is 112 pounds at 5'1" tall. At this point, I still did not understand that I was in a state of paranoid schizophrenia. I believed I was suffering from severe anxiety.

Before going on to chapter two which details the steps I took to get medical help for depression and schizophrenia, I would like to review the gifts I have mentioned throughout this chapter because I believe they were helpful in preparing me for the long road ahead to recovery.

MY GIFTS

1. Learning to play the piano
2. Learning to practice yoga
3. My Grandmother, Luella Abbott
4. My intelligence
5. My brother, Steven Duke
6. Learning to meditate

7. My Aunt Juanita Ingalls
8. The great outdoors
9. My best friend, Mary Krening
10. My mother, Helen Duke

Since this is a book that has been written to help others who may or may not be suffering from mental illness, an opportunity is now provided for the reader to reflect on his or her own life and identify the wonderful gifts that have helped you along the way. Take some time now to identify those people, places, or experiences that have been most helpful to you in dealing with the stresses of your life and write them in the Reader's Workbook which follows. If possible, identify why and how they have been gifts to you as well. Think about those people, places, or experiences that have provided you with opportunities for unconditional love, self-confidence, success, involvement in community, creativity, spiritual growth, accomplishment of your life's mission, etc.

READER'S WORKBOOK: YOUR GIFTS

1. _____

Why or how has this been a gift?

_____

_____

_____

_____

_____

_____

2. _____

Why or how has this been a gift?

_____

_____

_____

_____

_____

_____

3. _____

Why or how has this been a gift?

_____

_____

_____

_____

_____

_____

_____

4. _____

Why or how has this been a gift?

_____

_____

_____

_____

_____

_____

5. _____

Why or how has this been a gift?

_____

_____

_____

_____

_____

_____

_____

6. _____

Why or how has this been a gift?

_____

_____

_____

_____

_____

_____

7. _____

Why or how has this been a gift?

_____

_____

_____

_____

_____

_____

8. _____

Why or how has this been a gift?

_____

_____

_____

_____

_____

_____

9. _____

Why or how has this been a gift?

_____

_____

_____

_____

_____

_____

10. _____

Why or how has this been a gift?

_____

_____

_____

_____

_____

_____

CHAPTER TWO

Diagnosis

B ecause I believed I was suffering from severe anxiety, I purchased a book by Bloomfield (1998) entitled *Healing Anxiety with Herbs*. The book recommended kava which calms the nerves, valerian which relieves anxiety and insomnia, and chamomile which also calms the nerves. Additionally, I tried the flower essence remedy of cherry plum which is used when one has fears of losing one's mind or of going crazy. None of these remedies supplied me with any relief. The "voices" continued and I was surviving on very little sleep.

One day, late in June of 1998, I was at my mother's house reading a magazine article about medical intuitives who have the ability to assist you in healing. By chance, one of the medical intuitives featured in the article lived nearby. Her name was Dr. Cay Randall-May. I called for a healing appointment and she was able to see me the next day. She performed an energy healing treatment on me and shared with me afterward that she felt I had a chemical imbalance as well as an emotional imbalance and advised me to get a medical checkup from my family practice doctor as soon as possible.

I immediately made an appointment with my family doctor who was able to see me the first week in July. As the appointment neared, however, I became so upset with the prospect of verbalizing to my doctor that I was "hearing voices," that I made the decision to write this information down and hand the paper to my doctor to read. After reading my note, he tried to reassure me by saying that this might be an isolated and brief incident. However, he referred me immediately to a psychiatrist. The symptom my doctor wrote on the referral was "auditory hallucinations." This was the first time I realized that this applied to me. My family doctor also gave me a prescription to help me sleep.

When I called to make the appointment with the psychiatrist, I became somewhat frightened when the receptionist/nurse asked, "Are the voices you are hearing telling you to harm yourself or others?" I told her no and, here, I should explain to the reader that the voices never told me to harm myself or others. They did, at times, say that *they* were going to hurt *me*. In particular, when I would hike near the family cabin and cross an old wooden bridge, they would say that they were going to push me off the bridge, and I remember sometimes having the physical sensation of being pushed although I never fell.

The psychiatrist was able to see me that very day and met with me for a three hour evaluation. The psychiatrist prescribed an antipsychotic medication to alleviate the voices. Originally, I had two voices in my head, but, after only a few days of taking the antipsychotic, one of the voices went away completely never to be heard from again.

I would like to take a moment here to explain that the auditory and hallucinatory voices I heard should not be confused with one's own inner voice of intuition or the voice of the higher self. These "voices" are completely different in that intuitive thoughts or thoughts from the higher self are positive and helpful. Auditory hallucinations are delusional, negative, derogatory, and self-deprecating. As Sass (1995) explains in his book *The Paradoxes of Delusion*, delusional thinking can be described as, "the far point of the trajectory of a consciousness turned in upon itself." It is as though the mind has waged war on itself.

For individuals with severe schizophrenia, the delusions are winning the war with the mind. As an example, normal minded people are, understandably, horrified when someone like Andrea Yates kills her five children because the "voices" told her to do so or, more recently, Jared Loughner, kills six people and injures numerous others in Tucson, Arizona, for no apparent reason, and, most recently, James Holmes, of the Colorado movie massacre, kills and terrorizes. But, as someone who has had "voices" most likely to a much lesser degree, I can completely understand why Andrea Yates, Jared Loughner, and James Holmes did what they did. In their minds which were deep in delusion, they had no other choice. I was fortunate in that I sought help fairly quickly and my "break from reality" was two to three weeks in duration at most. However, Andrea Yates, Jared Loughner, and James Holmes may have had much longer "breaks from reality" which, as we can all agree, led to disaster.

It is so very important that more attention be paid by family members, teachers, and friends to inappropriate or unusual behaviors displayed very early on by those such as Andrea Yates, Jared Loughner, James Holmes, and others so that proper evaluations, therapy, medications, as well as other interventions can be made that might prevent such disasters. I believe we, as a society, have "dropped the ball" when it comes to monitoring our children's behaviors and helping them become responsible, social, peaceful, and contributing members of society. Some parents, especially, have "thrown up their hands" and "caved in" to the ideas of 1) allowing their children to spend inordinate amounts of time on the computer, playing video games, texting, and, otherwise, interacting primarily with machines and electronics rather than having face to face human contact, thus, reducing their ability to socialize, empathize, and "read" others' feelings, 2) allowing their children to attend "virtual schools" or take online classes rather than learn and practice the hard work of in class participation and cooperation, 3) not requiring their children to do chores at home to earn allowances or work part time jobs to learn how to earn money, budget, successfully and respectfully work for a boss, and save money for college, and 4) completely neglecting the spiritual and emotional needs of their children. I am not implying that all parents are guilty of this. Understandably, with today's economy, more and more parents work longer and harder hours and do not have as much time to devote to their children. But, I do continue to hear of so many instances where teachers, other family members, or friends have approached parents with serious concerns regarding their children's behaviors only to be ignored.

Our state and federal governments have reduced precious funding for helping those who are mentally ill. Mental illness continues to be a highly stigmatizing label. When someone shares that they have diabetes or cancer, a sympathetic shoulder is usually offered. Not so with mental illness which continues to be viewed with suspicion or shunned altogether. Perhaps the tragedies described above could have been avoided if society and our state and federal governments were more responsive and compassionate rather than judgmental and isolating to those suffering from mental illness.

There is still so much that we do not know about the causes of mental illness which may include genetics, chemical imbalances, hormonal imbalances, stress, isolation, low self-esteem, etc. Many people with mental illness suffer in silence with symptoms such as auditory hallucinations never telling anyone, not even family members, for fear they will be judged as "crazy." They attempt to hide the symptoms for as long as possible or until the symptoms escalate into severe paranoia and/or a life devastating breakdown. It may be surprising to the reader to learn that the majority of people with schizophrenia do not even know they have it. According to the National Alliance on Mental Illness (NAMI), "research studies have shown that over 50% of those living with schizophrenia do not believe themselves to be ill. This lack of awareness or insight is known as *anosognosia.*" In these cases, family members and others close to the person displaying the symptoms of schizophrenia must intervene to try and get help for the individual. This can be a fulltime job for family members, friends, and caretakers who constantly try to motivate and bring insight to the loved one in order to facilitate recovery from the mental illness. Getting help for the symptoms of schizophrenia, depression, anxiety, manic-depression, or any other mental illness must be pursued by either the individual who is suffering or through help by others. I was fortunate because I *knew* something was wrong and I wanted to get help fairly soon after my symptoms appeared.

In addition to prescribing antipsychotic medication, my psychiatrist ordered several blood tests and an MRI (magnetic resonance imaging) test which is a brain imaging technique that shows the brain in action. As I drove to the laboratory for my first-ever series of MRI scans, I remember hoping that the results would show that I had a brain tumor because I thought a brain tumor might be operable possibly leading to the elimination of the other "voice" in my head. The results turned out to be negative except for an indication of unusually high activity in the deep white matter of the brain (wherever or whatever that is). In short, my brain structure and functioning were normal. I was still unaware that I had been diagnosed with schizophrenia, but I knew I needed to get rid of this other "voice" somehow.

During the two weeks between my initial meeting with the psychiatrist and my next appointment, I fully expected that the antipsychotic medication would make the other voice go away. After about a week, I called the psychiatrist to inform him that the other voice had not gone away. He replied that the medication might take a little while to get into my system and take effect and he said we would talk more about it at our next appointment. In the meantime, although I was still on summer vacation, I worked on creating lesson plans so that I would be better prepared for teaching school which was scheduled to begin in the middle of August. I also purposely kept in contact with a couple of family members and one close friend. I was so very, very fortunate to have a job to go back to. Again, I must stress that I had what I would call an unusually mild case of schizophrenia. There are so many individuals, especially males, who develop the disorder in their late teens and early twenties before they have had a chance to complete high school and college, establish a career, get married, begin a family, etc. Consequently, because these individuals have not yet "begun their lives," they may feel they do not have much to lose or get back to. Needless to say, parents end up continuing to be caregivers of these adult children.

During my second visit with my psychiatrist, he decided to increase the dosage of the antipsychotic. Again, I believed this would lead to the elimination of the other voice. The antipsychotic was helpful in allowing me to sleep and the voice did seem to stay away most of the time. But, for several hours of each day, the voice would intrude with negative statements and commentary about me. Again, I tried to stay busy. I applied at another couple of universities for teaching positions. I did more schoolwork, lessons, and additional planning for school as well as cleaning at home. I tried hard to maintain a normal schedule. And, again, I called the psychiatrist to inform him that the voice had still not gone away. He again said we would talk about it further at our next session. The time between sessions two and three was three weeks.

At our third session, the doctor informed me that he believed my auditory hallucinations had been precipitated by depression and thought it would be helpful if I were to begin taking an antidepressant medication in addition to the antipsychotic. I, of course, agreed. It was not until six weeks later, at our next session, that I had the courage to ask the psychiatrist what my diagnosis was. He looked at me as if I should already know that it was schizophrenia with depression. I asked him how many cases of schizophrenia he had treated in his career. His reply was "somewhere between 800 and 1000 cases." I then asked him how many of those "cases" were ever able to be rid of the voices altogether. He thought for a moment and told me, "four or five." I was shocked. It was at this point that the idea began to set in that I may have these unwanted "voices" intruding on my life until the day I die.

DEALING WITH THE DIAGNOSIS

In dealing with the dual diagnoses of schizophrenia and depression, I believe I experienced all of the stages of grief that one experiences after the death of a loved one. I experienced denial where I felt that this just could not be true. It could not possibly be happening to me. No one else in my family had schizophrenia, so how could I possibly develop it? I do believe that feelings of depression were widespread within my family, but not schizophrenia. Next, I began to feel anger towards God, primarily. Why would God allow this to happen to me? I had always tried so hard to be good and do well for myself and the world. I was mad. I think I dealt with the anger by working harder at school and trying not to pay so much attention to God.

My anger soon ended and I began to accept my plight. What helped me the most in accepting the illnesses was remembering something my Grandmother Abbott used to say: "Things could always be worse." I had to agree. I was not in a wheelchair. I did not have cancer. I was not in prison. I did not require hospitalization. I had a fulltime job. I had a beautiful condominium to live in. I had a few family members and friends close by. I could still go hiking if I wanted to and practice my yoga. I even began to be thankful that there were medications available to help treat the schizophrenia and the depression. I was thankful that I had a good psychiatrist. Making it a habit to be in gratitude for all of the things I had going for me was the first step in my recovery. Whether you have schizophrenia, depression, any type of mental illness, or not, I believe this strategy would be helpful to anyone. It may be a strategy you already use. And, I believe that making it a daily habit will have a positive and healing effect on your life. Every morning, think about ten great things that could possibly happen for you today. Write them down. Then, at the end of the day, list ten wonderful things that either did happen or that you are grateful for. Take time right now to list ten wonderful things that you are either grateful for or that were positive in your life today.

READER'S WORKBOOK: THINGS TO BE GRATEFUL FOR

1. _____

_____

2. _____

_____

3. _____

_____

4. _____

_____

5. _____

_____

6. _____

_____

7. _____

_____

8. _____

_____

9. _____

_____

10. _____

_____

Before I go on to detail more fully my treatment and recovery processes in the following chapters, I would like to take time here to briefly educate the reader on the specific disorders of schizophrenia and depression. While I am absolutely no expert, I am a natural born researcher and completed both a thesis and a dissertation in education. I became very interested in finding out more about these illnesses including their definitions, symptoms, prevalence, treatments, and chances for recovery. To begin, think of any experience you have had up to this point in your life with schizophrenia and/or depression. What do you know about them? Do you, yourself, suffer from either or both disorders? Do you have family members or friends who have suffered from either of these mental illnesses? Take time right now to write a brief paragraph explaining what you know about schizophrenia and depression.

WHAT I KNOW ABOUT SCHIZOPHRENIA

_____

_____

_____

_____

_____

_____

_____

_____

_____

_____

_____

_____

_____

_____

_____

WHAT I KNOW ABOUT DEPRESSION

To help the average reader who has not studied schizophrenia or depression, I have included in this chapter two true false quizzes. First, take the quiz on schizophrenia and check your answers on the pages that follow. Then, do the same with the quiz on depression. All of the factual information provided has been taken from the NAMI (National Alliance on Mental Illness) website and from the book by Rosalynn Carter entitled *Helping Someone with Mental Illness* which was published in 1998. Other books I have studied to educate myself more fully on the topics of the brain and schizophrenia include Carper's *Your Miracle Brain*, Gray's *Gray's Anatomy*, and Marohn's *The Natural Guide to Schizophrenia*. They are listed in the references.

QUIZ ON SCHIZOPHRENIA

Answer true or false:

1. Schizophrenia is a brain disorder that affects approximately 2.4 million American adults, or 1.1 percent of the population aged 18 and older.

    True   False

2. A person with schizophrenia has a "split personality."

    True   False

3. Almost all people with schizophrenia are NOT dangerous or violent towards others when they are receiving treatment.

    True   False

4. Schizophrenia does not affect an individual's thinking or cognition.

    True   False

5. Schizophrenia seems to be caused by a combination of problems including genetic vulnerability and environmental factors.

    True   False

6. There is no cure for schizophrenia.

    True   False

7. The World Health Organization has identified schizophrenia as one of the ten most debilitating diseases affecting human beings.

True   False

8. No one symptom positively identifies schizophrenia.

True   False

9. Males are more likely to suffer from schizophrenia than females.

True   False

10. Males are more likely to develop schizophrenia when they are young while females tend to develop schizophrenia when they are older.

True   False

11. In the brain, the *thalamus,* which helps us filter, process, and relay input from our senses, emotions, and memory, is, on average, larger in people with schizophrenia than in the rest of the population.

True   False

12. The disease of schizophrenia is inherited.

True   False

13. The brains of people with schizophrenia have too much *dopamine,* a chemical neurotransmitter.

True   False

14. The symptoms of schizophrenia are generally divided into three categories including positive, disorganized, and negative symptoms.

True   False

15. People with schizophrenia require hospitalization at some point in their lives.

True   False

ANSWERS TO QUIZ ON SCHIZOPHRENIA

1. Schizophrenia is a brain disorder that affects approximately 2.4 million American adults, or 1.1 percent of the U.S. population aged 18 and older.

   True. One in every one hundred adults in America has schizophrenia.

2. A person with schizophrenia has a "split personality."

   False. A person with schizophrenia does not have a split personality. This is a common misconception due to the fact that the prefix *schizo* means "to split."

3. Almost all people with schizophrenia are NOT dangerous or violent towards others when they are receiving treatment.

   True. With proper treatment including therapy and medication, almost all people with schizophrenia are not dangerous or violent towards others or themselves.

4. Schizophrenia does not affect an individual's thinking or cognition.

   False. Some symptoms manifested by those with schizophrenia include confused thinking and speech and behavior that does not make sense. For example, people with schizophrenia sometimes have trouble communicating in coherent sentences or carrying on conversations with others. They may have difficulty making sense of everyday sights and sounds.

5. Schizophrenia seems to be caused by a combination of problems including genetic vulnerability and environmental factors.

   True. Compelling scientific evidence points to the fact that schizophrenia may be caused to a substantial degree by a combination of defects that occur early in the brain's development as a result of genetic vulnerability plus environmental triggers that may be quite physical in nature.

6. There is no cure for schizophrena.

   True and False. The National Association for Mental Illness (NAMI) reports that, while there is no cure for schizophrenia, it is a highly treatable and manageable disease. For many people with schizophrenia, I believe a cure might not be possible or likely. However, I am living proof that someone previously diagnosed with schizophrenia can be completely cured. I have no symptoms, I no longer receive therapy, and I am no longer on any medication. Therefore, I believe this statement is true for some individuals but false for others because I believe my case was not as severe as many who are diagnosed with the disease.

7. The World Health Organization has identified schizophrenia as one of the ten most debilitating diseases affecting human beings.

    True. Schizophrenia is one of the ten most debilitating diseases affecting human beings resulting, many times, in institutionalization, unemployment, poverty, homelessness, and imprisonment.

8. No one symptom positively identifies schizophrenia.

    True. All of the symptoms of schizophrenia can also be found in other brain disorders. For example, psychotic symptoms may be caused by the use of drugs, may be present in individuals with Alzheimer's Disease, or can manifest during a manic episode in a bipolar disordered individual. A doctor will usually analyze a patient's symptoms as well as carefully assess the history and the course of events over several months before making a diagnosis of schizophrenia.

9. Males are more likely to suffer from schizophrenia than are females.

    False. Males and females suffer from schizophrenia fairly equally. However, the age of onset of the disorder differs between males and females.

10. Males are more likely to develop schizophrenia when they are young while females tend to develop schizophrenia when they are older.

True. Males have an early onset usually between the ages of their late teens and twenties and females are more likely to have a later onset usually after age 30. My onset was at approximately age 41 or 42. While I have read no supportive research, I, personally, believe that a change in my hormones related to pre-menopause may have contributed to my development of the disorder. However, I have read research indicating that, due to the earlier onset of the illness for males, their lives are usually more debilitated by schizophrenia resulting in the homelessness, unemployment, poverty, institutionalization, and imprisonment mentioned earlier. I believe you are at an advantage to overcome schizophrenia if you are female.

11. In the brain, the *thalamus,* which helps us filter, process, and relay input from our senses, emotions, and memory, is, on average, larger in people with schizophrenia than in the rest of the population.

     False. The *thalamus,* which helps us filter, process, and relay input from our senses, emotions, and memory, is, on average, **smaller,** in people with schizophrenia. A person with a defective thalamus is likely to be flooded with information and overwhelmed with stimuli.

12. The disease of schizophrenia is inherited.

     False. What is inherited is not the disease itself but a predisposition for developing it, much like inheriting a risk for diabetes, alcoholism, or heart disease. The genes (and many genes are involved) set the stage so that an environmental "insult" such as low oxygen or a viral infection in the womb might lead to the defects in brain development that lead to schizophrenia.

13. The brains of people with schizophrenia have too much *dopamine,* a chemical neurotransmitter.

     True. In addition to the overproduction of dopamine, it is also believed that the dopamine signal is not being "decoded" properly. I know, specifically, that the antipsychotic medication I took works to block the neurotransmitters and receptors responsible for the re-uptake of dopamine. The medication also blocks other neurotransmitters and receptors throughout the body such as those in the stomach that communicate to the brain that you are "full." Because these neurotransmitters are blocked, the person taking the medication keeps eating because the brain has not received the message of being full. Therefore, a common side effect of taking certain antipsychotics is weight gain.

14. The symptoms of schizophrenia are generally divided into three categories including positive, disorganized, and negative symptoms.

> **True.** Positive symptoms include delusions and hallucinations because the patient has lost touch with reality in important ways. Positive does not mean "good." Rather, it refers to having overt symptoms that should not be there. Delusions cause patients to believe that people are monitoring their thoughts or plotting against them, or that they themselves control other people's minds. Hallucinations refer to the things people hear or see that are not there. Disorganized symptoms include those mentioned previously in quiz item four such as confused thinking and incoherent speech. Negative symptoms include emotional flatness or lack of expression, an inability to start and follow through with activities, speech that is brief and without emotion, a lack of pleasure or interest in life. "Negative," does not, therefore, refer to a bad attitude, but to a lack of certain characteristics that should be there.

15. People with schizophrenia require hospitalization at some point in their lives.

> **False.** While many with schizophrenia find themselves in and out of hospitals or institutions throughout their lives, I am living proof that one can develop the illness and be diagnosed with the disorder without ever requiring hospitalization. Others require hospitalization early on, and, with proper treatment including therapy and medication, require no further hospitalization in their lifetimes.

At this point, the reader might wish to take a break from reading in order to allow the information on schizophrenia to sink in and process. The reader may wish to highlight, star, or underline certain facts described in the quiz answers that are most helpful and enlightening to him or her, and, again, pause for a while before taking the quiz on depression that follows.

QUIZ ON DEPRESSION

Answer true or false:

1. Major depression is a serious mental illness affecting 15 million American adults, approximately 5 to 8 percent of the adult population in a given year.

                   True   False

2. More than twice as many women as men suffer from depression each year.

                   True   False

3. Left untreated, depression can lead to suicide.

                   True   False

4. In order to be diagnosed with depression, an individual must demonstrate all of the following symptoms: persistently sad or irritable mood, pronounced changes in sleep, appetite, and energy, difficulty thinking, concentrating, and remembering, physical slowing or agitation, lack of interest in or pleasure from activities that were once enjoyed, feelings of guilt, worthlessness, hopelessness, emptiness, recurrent thoughts of death or suicide, and persistent physical symptoms that do not respond to treatment, such as headaches, digestive disorders, and chronic pain.

                   True   False

5. Scientific research has firmly established that major depression is a psychological disorder.

                   True   False

6. Norepinephrine, serotonin, and dopamine are three neurotransmitters (chemical messengers that transmit electrical

signals between brain cells) that are believed to be out of balance, thus resulting in clinical depression.

True   False

7. The disorder of depression is inherited.

True   False

8. Seventy-five percent of those suffering from severe depression can be effectively treated and return to their normal daily activities and feelings.

True   False

9. There are three basic types of treatment for depression: medication, psychotherapy, and electroconvulsive therapy (ECT).

True   False

10. The risk of suicide may temporarily increase when a patient with depression is first placed on antidepressant medication.

True   False

11. Researchers believe that increased amounts of serotonin and other neurotransmitters produced in the brain are involved in depression, causing the sleep problems, irritability, anxiety, fatigue, and despondent mood that characterize the illness.

True   False

12. Decreased serotonin activity in the brain may be linked to suicidal behavior.

True   False

13. Depressed people experience normal sleep cycles.

True   False

14. The most common and effective treatment for severely depressed individuals is a combination of psychotherapy and antidepressant medication.

True   False

15. A person diagnosed with depression must remain on antidepressant medication for the rest of his or her lifetime.

True   False

ANSWERS TO QUIZ ON DEPRESSION

1. Major depression is a serious mental illness affecting 15 million American adults, approximately 5 to 8 percent of the adult population in a given year.

    True. Major depression affects 15 million American adults, approximately 5-8 percent of the adult population.

2. More than twice as many women as men suffer from depression each year.

    True. More than twice as many women (10 million) as men (5 million) suffer from depression each year. Major depression can occur at any age including the teenage years and adulthood. All ethnic, racial, and socioeconomic groups suffer from depression. About three-fourths of those who experience a first episode of depression have at least one other episode in their lives.

3. Left untreated, depression can lead to suicide.

    True. However, men commit suicide four times as often as women do. It is theorized that women, when considering suicide, are more likely to get help from medical professionals than men.

4. In order to be diagnosed with depression, an individual must demonstrate all of the following symptoms: persistently sad or irritable mood, pronounced changes in sleep, appetite, and energy, difficulty thinking, concentrating, and remembering, physical slowing or agitation, lack of interest in or pleasure from activities that were once enjoyed, feelings of guilt, worthlessness, hopelessness, emptiness, recurrent thoughts of death or suicide, and persistent physical symptoms that do not respond to treatment, such as headaches, digestive disorders, and chronic pain.

    False. An individual need not exhibit all of the symptoms of depression. When several of these symptoms occur at the same time for longer than two weeks, and interfere with ordinary functioning, professional treatment for depression is needed.

5. Scientific research has firmly established that major depression is a psychological disorder.

   False. There is no single cause of major depression. Psychological, biological, and even environmental factors may contribute to its development. Whatever the specific causes of depression, scientific research has firmly established that major depression is a **biological** disorder.

6. Norepinephrine, serotonin, and dopamine are three neurotransmitters (chemical messengers that transmit electrical signals between brain cells) that are believed to be out of balance, thus resulting in clinical depression.

   True. Scientists believe that if there is a chemical imbalance among neurotransmitters, then clinical states of depression result. Antidepressant medications work by increasing the availability of neurotransmitters or by changing the receptors for these chemical messengers.

7. The disorder of depression is inherited.

   False. Scientists have found evidence of a genetic predisposition to major depression. There is also an increased risk for developing depression if there is a family history of depression. However, not everyone with a genetic predisposition develops depression, but some people probably have a biological make-up that leaves them particularly vulnerable to developing the disorder. Life events, such as the death of a loved one, a major loss or life change, stress, and alcohol and drug abuse, may trigger episodes of depression. It is also important to note that many depressive episodes occur spontaneously and are not triggered by a life crisis, physical illness, or other risks.

8. Seventy-five percent of those suffering from severe depression can be effectively treated and return to their normal daily activities and feelings.

False. Although major depression can be a devastating illness, it is highly treatable. Between **85 and 90 percent** of those suffering from severe depression can be effectively treated and return to their normal daily activities and feelings.

9. There are three basic types of treatment for depression: medication, psychotherapy, and electroconvulsive therapy (ECT).

    True. Medication, psychotherapy, and electroconvulsive therapy (ECT) may be used singly or in combination. Medications include *tricyclic antidepressants* (TCAs) still widely used for severe depression to elevate mood in depressed individuals and to re-establish their normal sleep and energy levels, *monoamine oxidase inhibitors* (MAOIs) which are often effective in individuals who do not respond to other medications or who have "atypical" depressions that include such symptoms as anxiety, excessive sleeping, irritability, hypochondria, or phobic characteristics, *selective serotonin reuptake inhibitors* (SSRIs) which act specifically on the neurotransmitter serotonin (in general, SSRIs cause fewer side effects than TCAs and MAOIs), *serotonin and norepinephrine reuptake inhibitors* (SNRIs) which are useful in treating people who are taking an antidepressant for the first time and for those who have not responded to other medications (in general, SNRIs cause fewer side effects than TCAs and MAOIs), and *bupropion* which is a newer antidepressant medication classified as a dopamine reuptake blocking compound. Mild to moderate depression can often be treated successfully with psychotherapy alone. Two predominating types of psychotherapy include *cognitive-behavioral therapy* (CBT) which helps to change the negative thinking and unsatisfying behavior associated with depression and to teach people how to unlearn the behavioral patterns that contribute to their illness and *interpersonal therapy* (IPT) which focuses on improving troubled personal relationships and on adapting to new life roles that may have been associated with a person's depression. Finally, *electroconvulsive therapy* (ECT) is a highly effective treatment for severe depressive episodes. In situations where medication, psychotherapy, and/or a combination of the two prove ineffective or work too slowly to relieve severe symptoms such as psychosis or thoughts of suicide, ECT may be considered. ECT can also be considered for those who for one reason or another cannot take antidepressant medications.

10. The risk of suicide may temporarily increase when a patient with depression is first placed on antidepressant medication.

    True. Consumers (those with depression) and their families must be cautious during the early stages of antidepressant treatment because normal energy levels and the ability to take action often improve before mood improves. At this time – when decisions are easier to make, because the depression is still severe – the risk of suicide may temporarily increase.

11. Researchers believe that increased amounts of serotonin and other neurotransmitters produced in the brain are involved in depression, causing the sleep problems, irritability, anxiety, fatigue, and despondent mood that characterize the illness.

    False. Researchers believe that **decreased** amounts of serotonin and other neurotransmitters produced in the brain are involved in depression, causing the sleep problems, irritability, anxiety, fatigue, and despondent mood that characterize the illness.

12. Decreased serotonin activity in the brain may be linked to suicidal behavior.

    True. Decreased serotonin activity in the brain may be linked to suicidal behavior. Autopsies of suicide victims have revealed lesser amounts of serotonin in the fluid surrounding the brain and spinal cord than is normal, and certain brain cells in these victims seem to have more receptors for serotonin, as if to make up for the inadequate supply.

13. Depressed people experience normal sleep cycles.

    False. The normal sleep pattern is made up of several ninety-minute cycles during the night with various stages of deeper sleep plus REM (rapid eye movement) sleep – an almost waking state in which dreams occur. For most of us, deep sleep occurs early in the night, with REM sleep being only a small fraction of the first ninety-minute cycle and taking up more time in the cycles as the night progresses. The pattern seems to reverse for depressed individuals. They experience long stretches of the more wakeful REM sleep early in the night and less toward morning. This sleep pattern may account for some of the exhaustion many depressed people feel when they wake up.

14. The most common and effective treatment for severely depressed individuals is a combination of psychotherapy and antidepressant medication.

    True. Psychotherapy and antidepressant medication reinforce each other – the psychotherapy puts those affected in a frame of mind that makes them more apt to stick to their medication schedule, and the medication puts them in the frame of mind that makes their therapy more beneficial.

15. A person diagnosed with depression must remain on antidepressant medication for the rest of his or her lifetime.

    False. As mentioned previously, those suffering from mild to moderate depression may be treated through psychotherapy alone. However, those with severe depression may need to take antidepressant medications throughout their lifetime.

Take a moment to highlight, star, or underline any interesting or useful information provided in the quiz answers and then return to your descriptions of what you know about schizophrenia and depression to see how your perceptions may have changed after taking the quizzes. The answers in these quizzes provide the basics. However, there has been and continues to be an extraordinary amount of information, research, and personal accounts available for your investigation. In the references and recommended reading section at the end of this book, you will find listed other books and resources that may be of interest and/or prove helpful. In the appendix, the reader will find many websites and further information on support groups and courses for those with mental illness and for those who are family members, friends, or caregivers of those with mental illness. Most of the entries in the appendix have been taken from the National Alliance on Mental Illness (NAMI) website. Recent research articles on a variety of mental illness topics and issues can also be found on the NAMI website.

In chapter three, I will provide details of the treatment I received for schizophrenia and depression during the years of 1998 and 1999 including medication side effects along with insights into the disorders which were greatly facilitated by my psychiatrist. I will also offer within the Reader's Workbook opportunities for reflection and goal setting for family members and caretakers of those with mental illness.

CHAPTER THREE

Treatment 1998-1999

B y the time I met with my psychiatrist again in late September of 1998, the school year was well underway. Throughout the school day, I was able to successfully perform my job duties as a teacher with no interference from the "voice." It seemed that if I kept my mind busy and focused, I was able to keep the voice away. I continued to give thanks daily for the strength in the medications that calmed my mind. I was also thankful that I was not in a hospital somewhere without a job. The "voice" continued to "intrude" outside of my work day, but its intrusions were what I would term "bearable." I no longer felt paranoid or as fearful. The "voice" became more of a nuisance.

Almost every time I visited my psychiatrist throughout the fall of 1998, he would increase the dosage of either the antipsychotic or the antidepressant. By spring of 1999, I was taking 20 milligrams of the antipsychotic and 225 milligrams of the antidepressant daily. I gained twenty pounds (a common side effect of this particular antipsychotic). I also suffered from severe constipation. My psychiatrist was very helpful in providing explanations for the side effects. As I mentioned in chapter two, certain antipsychotics block neurotransmitters and receptors throughout the body (not just in the brain) such as those in the stomach that communicate to the brain that one is "full." Because these neurotransmitters and receptors were blocked, I would continue eating because my brain had not received the message that I was full.

My psychiatrist advised me to measure out my portions more carefully and eat only those portions. I also believe that the higher dosage of the antipsychotic required me to sleep about eleven hours each night. Sometimes, I would eat dinner at 6:00pm and go to sleep at 6:30pm. I would then awaken at 5:30am in order to get ready for work. For the constipation, the doctor recommended I take extra magnesium which has the effect of speeding up the digestion process. The magnesium provided magnificent relief and I recommended its use to other members of my family who suffered from constipation periodically even though they were not taking antipsychotic medications.

During the fall of 1998, I developed a "mask like" or "dead" expression on my face. This is another common side effect of certain antipsychotic medications. I remember looking at photographs taken during Christmastime while I was visiting family in Florida and I could clearly see this "mask like, dead" expression on my face in the photos. It seemed there was not enough make-up available to "cheer" up my face.

Because I had gained weight, I forced myself to join a hiking class which met on Saturdays during October and November of 1998. This was good because it forced me to get back out into the community. It had become too easy to relax into a daily life of working, eating, and sleeping. In retrospect, I believe that taking all of those medications had robbed me of my zest for life. I remember reading as a teenager, that drinking alcohol "consumed" the spirit. I think the same can be said for antipsychotics and antidepressants, at least in my case. While I marvel at the success these medications have in reducing the paranoia, allowing one to relax, and helping one not to be obsessed with one's problems, I believe there has to come a time when the true problems must be identified and addressed. A person could, theoretically and practically, spend the rest of his or her life on the medications never addressing the underlying causes of the illness. It can be an "easy" way out for some people since it can require great effort to overcome and grow from issues that may have caused the illness in the first place.

As stated earlier in chapter two, most people afflicted with schizophrenia and/or depression respond most favorably to treatment that combines medication and psychotherapy. The psychotherapy portion of the treatment is the place where the psychiatrist and patient together can begin to address the underlying causes of the illness. I was fortunate because I had a psychiatrist who helped me become knowledgeable about the illnesses I faced and took the time to talk about my problems. He would also offer suggestions for becoming more connected and involved in my community.

When I went to a session with my psychiatrist I could count on two things: 1) spending a good 45-60 minutes with him, and 2) waiting to see him for sometimes up to 60 minutes because he was spending so much time with the previous patient(s). But, I never faulted him for this. I believe it is safe to say that far too many psychiatrists spend only the required 15 to 20 minutes with each patient and much of that time is used in the discussion of how the medication is affecting the patient and what the next prescription and/or dosage should be. I further believe that more patients suffering from schizophrenia and depression would be able to function with lower dosages of the medications or without them completely if their therapy sessions were more intense and fruitful.

Two of the most beneficial pieces of information my psychiatrist ever shared with me were that individuals best able to deal with the illness of schizophrenia have: 1) logical insight into the disorder, and 2) a high self-esteem. As I will share more fully in chapter four, when I began to get a handle on where my self-esteem was and how I could improve it, I began to make great strides in overcoming both schizophrenia and depression.

By the end of 1998, the school year was nearly half over. I was on high dosages of medications for the schizophrenia and depression and receiving ongoing psychotherapy from my psychiatrist. Even though I was doing "okay," I dared not tell anyone at work that I had either of these illnesses. Schizophrenia, in particular, is an illness that many people do not understand. I worried that if someone in my workplace was to find out, then I might no longer be employed. Here I was, educated with a master's degree as well as a doctoral degree, in my twentieth year of successful teaching, and I was terrified that I might lose my job. Fortunately, I had several family members and one friend with whom I confided my diagnoses. They were extremely supportive and for that I will be eternally grateful. Still, my feelings of safety and security were compromised due to the fact that I believed I might lose employment because of the stigma and misunderstanding related to the word "schizophrenia." I went through a period of time where I was hard on myself and felt guilty for not being strong enough to avoid this illness. I realize now that this kind of thinking was and is completely unproductive. But, at the time, those feelings of not being good enough were entirely real for me. Again, I would like to reiterate here the need for compassion, non-judgment, and understanding towards those who suffer from mental illness. Even with the current stigma attached to labels such as schizophrenia, bipolar disorder, and even depression and obsessive compulsive disorder, the ability to recover can be further delayed due to an individual's loss of self-esteem and worry regarding being perceived as not good enough nor accepted by society.

Even though I was earning the highest salary of my teaching career, I took a part time job as an adjunct faculty member teaching for a local university in order to earn extra money. I taught a couple of classes each semester online and via correspondence to masters level education students. This was highly interesting to me. After twenty years of teaching elementary school, it was refreshing and different to work with university students. All of this work I was able to do from home via computer, mail, and telephone. It was helpful to me to be communicating one on one with university students who were also current teachers working on their masters' degrees. I was able to share in the successes they were having in their classrooms and this gave me a great feeling of purpose and of fulfilling my mission in life. I taught masters level courses online and via correspondence for four years. I was highly motivated and gained a good deal of self-confidence in my ability to teach and work at the university level.

Back in chapter one, you will recall that I identified and elaborated on ten "gifts" I had received throughout my lifetime and how they had helped me. Many of them continued to be helpful to me as I progressed through the early months of adjusting to my diagnoses and medications. For instance, I continued to practice yoga, however infrequently, and meditated periodically. Using these two gifts helped me to remember my spirit and my soul in spite of all the medications I was taking. My intelligence continued to serve as a gift to me in that it enabled me to begin researching schizophrenia and depression. My intelligence also supported me in the part time university work I was performing. My brother, Steve, my mother, other family members, and my best friend, Mary, continued to provide much needed support.

From July, 1998, until May, 1999, I noticed other "gifts" that came into my life. One of these was my good fortune in securing an outstanding psychiatrist. I do not believe I would have made the progress I have made in as speedy a manner had I not had in my life this medical professional, Dr. H. Lee Mitchell. Another gift was my part time job at the university.

As I just mentioned, my self-confidence was greatly enhanced and I was forced to interact with and support my students. The part time position helped to lift me out of my daily routine of teaching elementary school, eating, and sleeping.

Throughout the spring of 1999, I began to realize that I was ready to end my twenty year elementary teaching career and look for more interesting employment. My twenty years of teaching were extremely rewarding, challenging, and fulfilling. I believe I made a difference in the lives of a great many children. I still wanted to do that, but in a different way. I had worked very hard to earn my doctoral degree and most who obtain this degree do not continue teaching in the public schools. Someone with a doctorate in education might go on to teach at a university, work at the state department of education, work as an administrator in the public schools, do educational consulting, or something else. I decided to become an educational consultant and continue my part time work at the university.

In August of 1999, I accepted my new position as an educational consultant for an education company that specialized in helping teachers and administrators improve student achievement. Our customer base included school districts from across the nation labeled as underperforming or behind academically. This meant that their achievement scores were low. Low academic achievement for a school or district occurs more frequently in high poverty areas where there are higher percentages of minority students including those who are learning to speak, read, and write English as a second language. Our company had developed a program designed to assist teachers in teaching more effectively in order to raise achievement scores. My job was to train administrators and teachers across the nation on our program as well as to provide follow-up consultation and evaluate their success in implementing the program. The schools I had taught in for twenty years were excellent, middle to upper class schools in Arizona. My new position as a consultant took me into high poverty, high minority areas such as rural Georgia and Alabama, Milwaukee, New Orleans, Sacramento, East St. Louis, the Bronx in New York, and inner city Los Angeles. I traveled to many other places as well. I learned an enormous amount and saw even more including extreme poverty, poor school facilities, and ineffective teachers holding low expectations for minority and impoverished students. Through this new job, I became an expert on language arts and mathematics curriculum and assessment in schools and I considered this new career another gift in my life.

Because our customers were scattered across the country, I also became an expert at traveling by plane and rental car. I learned to deeply appreciate those who must travel for a living because it can be difficult, tiring, boring, and monotonous. During the first three months of my new job, I went on fifteen trips of two to five days each. I was really racking up the frequent flyer miles! More difficult than the flying, however, was trying to find the school where I was scheduled to conduct my in-service trainings. I am now an expert map reader and mapquester. This was before the widespread use of electronic navigation systems! Even though my travel schedule was hectic, I continued with my medication regimen and visits to the psychiatrist. The "voice" was still there, at times, but, I believe I was so busy that it did not get much time to intrude. I was still sleeping a great deal. Because I was "on the road" so much, I was unable to exercise as regularly and gained still more weight. During this time, however, it seemed I was able to feel a little more balanced in my life. When I was at home, I would take more time to schedule social activities with friends and family. I would also take time on weekends to travel up to our family's cabin to squeeze in a hike here and there. I think it is extremely important that anyone diagnosed with schizophrenia and/or depression stay busy working, reading, exercising, taking classes, etc. in order to support the mind in functioning productively. I also believe it is imperative that any individual suffering from mental illness remain social even if "by force" from family members, friends, and caretakers. I seemed to intuitively understand that staying busy and remaining social would be strong building blocks to my recovery. If these actions do not regularly occur, then a mentally ill individual is left to him or herself feeling isolated, nonproductive, and with time on his or her hands to interact with the voices, create new voices in their heads to have conversations with, or, as in the case of depression, become even further depressed. I concluded that the more one isolates oneself, the more likely it would be that future "breaks from reality" would occur. I did not want to ever have another "break from reality," so I decided to get busy, stay involved, take classes, and learn new skills that would help me to heal and stay balanced.

In November of 1999, I registered to take a class on Reiki (a healing art) that met for two weeks on Saturday mornings. This particular type of Reiki was in the Usui tradition and the reader is invited to research this particular type of Reiki. Taking this class proved to be another incredible gift for me in that it started me down this long road I have taken to heal and become whole. Reiki is a form of energetic healing that is transmitted through the hands and assists in establishing optimal energy flow throughout the body. The class I attended in 1999 was an introductory course. In the next chapter, I will describe the training I received in Mahatma Reiki and how I began to use Reiki to heal my own body and mind.

Allow me to take a moment here to review the additional gifts that came into my life during the first eighteen months of my treatment after having been diagnosed with schizophrenia and depression. I mention these because I believe finding gifts in one's life even when things look bleak is an important strategy to use in order to feel hope, joy, and gratitude.

MORE GIFTS

1. The medical intuitive, Dr. Cay Randall-May
2. Full time teaching position
3. Lovely home I owned
4. NAMI (National Alliance on Mental Illness)
5. Medications (antidepressants and antipsychotics)
6. Part time university teaching position
7. Continued support of family and friends
8. My psychiatrist, Dr. H. Lee Mitchell
9. New career as an educational consultant
10. Introduction to Usui Reiki

At this point, I would like to invite the reader to take a look back at his or her own life to a time when you experienced a severe setback in the form of either an illness you or a family member was diagnosed with, a breakup or divorce, a bankruptcy, or some other crisis in your life that was very stressful and/or debilitating to you. A special invitation is made here to the families and friends of mental illness sufferers. Having to guide, take care of, and support family members diagnosed with a mental illness including the elderly who are increasingly being diagnosed with Alzheimers can be very energy depleting and hopeless. Steps most certainly must be taken by these dear and selfless caregivers to find support for themselves so they can achieve a balanced life that includes fun, relationships, friends, travel, hobbies, and good health. Caregivers must be willing to reach out for this help and support for themselves. I believe in the old yet applicable adage that one is better able to give to others if one takes care of oneself first. Remember? On the airplane? Put your own oxygen mask on before helping others with theirs ☺

Back to the current workbook exercise: think about what was going on in your life when you were 15, 20, 25, 30, 35, etc. to help you recall. Name several of those setbacks:

READER'S WORKBOOK: MAJOR SETBACKS IN YOUR LIFE

1. _____

_____

2. _____

_____

3. _____

_____

4. _____

_____

5. _____

_____

6. _____

_____

7. _____

_____

8. _____

_____

9. _____

_____

10. _____

_____

Now, review the list and circle the number of the one that was most difficult for you. Next, you will have the opportunity to write about why this setback was so hard. This is a four part assignment (you can tell I am a teacher:). In the first paragraph, write only about the feelings you went through in response to this setback. In the second paragraph, describe how this setback affected your life at home, at work, socially, spiritually, physically, and in any other way you can think of. In the third paragraph, explain how you managed to cope or get through the setback. Be specific and try to think of several strategies you used. In the fourth paragraph, identify any gifts that emerged as a result of living through the setback, crisis, or loss. Gifts can take many forms. Maybe you made a new friend or you focused more attention on getting healthy physically. Perhaps you tapped back into your own spirituality. Take your time and try to focus on the early stages or months subsequent to the setback, crisis, or loss.

MOST DIFFICULT SETBACK IN YOUR LIFE

Write the most difficult setback below:

_____

_____

_____

_____

_____

_____

_____

How did you feel?

_____

_____

_____

_____

_____

_____

_____

_____

_____

_____

_____

_____

_____

_____

_____

How did the setback affect you?

How did you cope?

_____

_____

_____

_____

_____

_____

_____

_____

_____

_____

_____

_____

_____

_____

What gifts emerged?

_____

_____

_____

_____

_____

_____

_____

_____

_____

_____

_____

_____

_____

_____

The purpose of this exercise was two-fold. First, I believe it is important to review how you dealt with a setback or crisis in the past in order to identify the tools you used to survive the ordeal. Some of the tools may have been healthy and some not so healthy. If you can recognize that you have within your own "coping toolbox" some healthy tools, perhaps they can continue to be applied in the present and in the future. The second purpose of the exercise was to identify and recognize that out of any setback emerge gifts that help us grow, learn, and become better human beings. I believe the gifts help us to become more closely aligned to our spirit and our mission in life. For myself, I believe it was this improved alignment with my own spirit and mission that led to my choice to no longer allow auditory hallucinations (the "voice") to intrude on my mind or my spirit. I will further explain this phenomenon in chapter four.

Before ending chapter three, however, I would like to present a Reader's Workbook section for family members, friends, and caregivers currently assisting those with mental illness.

READER'S WORKBOOK: CURRENT FAMILY MEMBERS, FRIENDS, AND CAREGIVERS

1. Who in your life are you currently caring for who is diagnosed with mental illness? Describe:

_____

_____

_____

_____

_____

_____

_____

_____

_____

_____

_____

_____

_____

2. For how long have you been providing care and assistance? Describe:

_____

_____

_____

_____

_____

_____

_____

_____

_____

_____

_____

_____

_____

_____

_____

3. Do you have anyone else in your life helping you to provide care? Describe:

---

4. What is the prognosis for your loved one regarding their mental illness? Describe:

_____

_____

_____

_____

_____

_____

_____

_____

_____

_____

_____

_____

_____

_____

_____

_____

5. What are your hopes for the individual for which you are caring?

6. What strategies are you currently using to help your mentally ill loved one move toward achieving these goals?

_____

_____

_____

_____

_____

_____

_____

_____

_____

_____

_____

_____

_____

_____

_____

_____

7. How has your work as a caretaker affected your life?

_____

_____

_____

_____

_____

_____

_____

_____

_____

_____

_____

_____

_____

_____

_____

_____

_____

8. Do you believe you currently have balance in your life? Explain.

_____

_____

_____

_____

_____

_____

_____

_____

_____

_____

_____

_____

_____

_____

_____

_____

9. What do you currently do to try to keep balance in your life?

_____

_____

_____

_____

_____

_____

_____

_____

_____

_____

_____

_____

_____

_____

_____

_____

10. **Are you, yourself, happy? If yes or no, explain:**

11. What do you do for fun, hobbies, travel, relationships, and friendships?

_____

_____

_____

_____

_____

_____

_____

_____

_____

_____

_____

_____

_____

_____

_____

_____

12. **What else could you do to bring more joy into your own life?**

_____

_____

_____

_____

_____

_____

_____

_____

_____

_____

_____

_____

_____

_____

_____

13. What else could you do to bring more joy into your mentally ill loved one's life?

_____

_____

_____

_____

_____

_____

_____

_____

_____

_____

_____

_____

_____

_____

_____

_____

CHAPTER FOUR

Treatment and Strategic Relief

Early in the year 2000, I began to communicate to my psychiatrist that the medications were too strong for me. He tried changing me to a different antipsychotic medication and a different antidepressant medication. Neither of the medications agreed with me at all and soon I returned to the original antipsychotic and antidepressant he had me on before. Because of all the changes in medications, I visited the psychiatrist nearly every month for the first six months of 2000. I was still somewhat resigned to the fact that I would need to be on these medications for the rest of my life in order to mask the schizophrenia and depression. I say "mask" because, while on the medications, nearly all of the symptoms of schizophrenia and depression were erased and replaced with side effects. Some of the side effects I have described already and included weight gain, constipation, and a "mask like or dead" expression on my face.

I decided to do more about the weight gain and joined an at-work Weight Watchers group. My mother had experienced success in losing weight with Weight Watchers many years ago. By most standards, I was not viewed as overweight. I weighed in at the first meeting at 130 pounds and wanted to reduce to 110 pounds. I had a nice wardrobe of clothes that I had grown out of but wanted to fit back into. The support group atmosphere encouraged me to interact with others more, become a better listener, and empathize with others' struggles with weight. Weight Watchers uses a point system which is basically a system for counting calories. Each point is worth approximately 50 calories. Therefore, if I wanted to lose weight steadily in order to trim down to 110 pounds, I needed to eat approximately 24 points worth of food every day. That would equal about 1200 calories. I am only 5'1" so I needed fewer calories than most. In Weight Watchers, you keep a journal of everything you eat and drink including their point values. You learn to measure out your food more carefully and become much more aware of portion sizes. For the reader's information, the Weight Watchers organization has a newer program that can be learned about online at www.WeightWatchers.com

For me, there were four keys to losing weight on Weight Watchers: 1) planning my next day's diet including point values that added up to 24 points, 2) writing down everything I ate for the day even if I "cheated" a little by eating something that was not planned and, therefore, going over on my points, 3) exercising every day, and 4) weighing myself every day. Weight Watchers is not a "quick fix" or "magic bullet." It took me ten months to lose the twenty pounds. But, by practicing these strategies every day for ten months, they became habits. They are now part of my lifestyle. I continue to use these four strategies every day and have maintained an eighteen to twenty pound weight loss for over ten years. I still go "over my points" on some days and gain a couple of pounds once in a while, but if I go back to my 24 points or lower rule and consistently exercise, then I shed those extra pounds.

I cannot say enough about how Weight Watchers has improved my life, health, and self-esteem. I just feel better about myself and my body image when I'm at my goal weight. My clothes fit better and I feel more attractive and successful. These feelings contribute to a higher self-esteem for me. I believe self-esteem is something that lies on a continuum from low to high. It is something that only I, as an individual, have the power to control. Maintaining a high self-esteem takes everyday effort. It is almost as if I must wake up every morning and fill myself up with self-esteem. I have learned over the years that I can do this by saying nice things to myself about my body, mind, and spirit. I have discovered the importance of thinking positive thoughts, and reading and saying positive affirmations to keep the mind happy. I once read a quote by Ernest Holmes, the founder of Science of Mind, which asserted "one must guard the mind as if it was a garden of beautiful flowers." That visual image has stayed with me and I work hard to guard my own mind from negative thinking and do all that I can to keep the flowers beautiful there.

It was this realization that I could control my own self-esteem as well as my own mind that allowed me to say goodbye to the auditory hallucination of the "voice" that was still in my mind as a result of the schizophrenia. Although it was still there, because of the medications it did not "rear its ugly head" very often. I began to notice that I would start to get an intuition that the voice was just about to say something before it actually did. When I got that feeling, I would immediately begin to sing a song in my head, think about a positive plan I had for the future, or remember a positive memory from my past. If I tried any of these three strategies, the "voice" would not come through. It was as though I could stop it from speaking. I did this for several months beginning in January, 2000. I was effectively able to stop the voice. I thought this was just miraculous! Someone suffering from schizophrenia must truly want to get rid of the voices in order to become mentally healthy. Because the mind has "turned in on itself," the sufferer needs to recreate and recapture the healthy mind. This involves making the choice to re-enter society, make friends, become educated, eat healthfully, exercise, explore interests, and follow one's dreams. If the individual has a low self-esteem, is lacking in interests, goals, and friends, then he or she may actually favor maintaining the voices which serve as distractions and friends for the schizophrenic to converse with. In some ways, it may feel "safer" for the person with schizophrenia to stay "stuck" with the voices for a very long time because it does take courage, strength, work, and an increased self-esteem and a sense of self-worth to motivate oneself to "want" to get rid of the voices.

I also believe that the longer an individual remains "out of touch" with reality or the more frequently the individual experiences "breaks from reality," the less likely it is that the schizophrenic will be able to fully recapture his or her own mind, get off of the medications, and/or lead a happy and fulfilling life. I do not wish for the reader to lose hope here. I still believe that full or partial recovery is possible. As I stated earlier, my case of schizophrenia was what I would term mild with only a two to three week span of time during which I was in severe paranoia and out of touch with reality. The keys are to get medical help right away and then begin the long road back to wholeness. It took me two years to get to the point where I was ready to "release" the unhealthy voice in my head altogether.

In May of 2000, I was on a beautiful hike up near our family's cabin when I came to the realization that my mind had the power to never hear from this "voice" again. It had taken a very long period of time during which I took medication, participated in ongoing cognitive behavioral therapy with my psychiatrist, read books, listened to music and purposely "interrupted" the voice when I sensed that it was just about to say something before I made it to this point where I truly believed I had the strength, willpower, angelic support, and healed spirit all combining to allow this miracle to occur for me in my life. I made a vow to myself right then and there that I would never hear this hallucinatory "voice" again for the rest of my life. And, again, with the continued mental strategies I had developed, prayers, positive thinking, and goal setting, I never have. It was as though I had decided to completely recapture my mind and guard it, as Ernest Holmes would say "like a garden." It was also at this time that I became even more in tune with my own spirit, soul, and purpose in life. I want to emphasize to the reader that this ability to release the voice from ever again being heard in my head by me was not an overnight sensation. It had taken close to two long years to get ready and be successful in achieving this.

As I mentioned, I realized that this would take daily and even hourly work and effort. I would need to continue doing all of the things I had been doing such as maintaining a high self-esteem, eating healthfully, exercising, meditating, doing yoga, continuing to learn and do my best at work, and continuing to reach out and interact with family and friends. But, the work would not end here. There was still so much more that I could do. Next, I will describe two other strategies that I learned and used to help me release the disorders of schizophrenia and depression even more. The first was learning how to heal myself using Mahatma Reiki and the second was volunteering at a local mental health agency in order to help and support others diagnosed with schizophrenia.

Before I go on to describe these additional strategies, I would like to provide you, the reader, an opportunity to take a look at your own self-esteem. Because a good self-esteem is fundamental to good mental health, it is worth taking the time to analyze the steps and strategies you utilize every day to promote and maintain a positive self-esteem. First, describe your feelings about yourself right at this moment. Is your self-esteem high, low, or somewhere in the middle? Then, explain why you think your self-esteem is where it is. Next, describe several strategies you personally use to improve and/or maintain your self-esteem. Do you use positive affirmations? Do you call a friend or talk to a family member and ask them to give you some positive feedback or words of encouragement? Finally, take a moment to think about two or three positive steps or actions you could take that you think might further improve your self-esteem and write them down. These may become goals for you later on.

READER'S WORKBOOK: YOUR SELF-ESTEEM

Describe your self-esteem as it feels right at this moment.

_____

_____

_____

_____

_____

_____

_____

_____

_____

_____

_____

_____

_____

_____

_____

_____

Why do you think your self-esteem is where it is?

_____

_____

_____

_____

_____

_____

_____

_____

_____

_____

_____

_____

_____

_____

What strategies do you use to improve your self-esteem?

_____

_____

_____

_____

_____

_____

_____

_____

_____

_____

_____

_____

_____

_____

_____

_____

What additional steps or actions could you take to further improve your self-esteem?

_____

_____

_____

_____

_____

_____

_____

_____

_____

_____

_____

_____

_____

_____

MAHATMA REIKI

After having taken a brief, introductory class on Usui Reiki, I combed the telephone book to find the name of someone who taught Reiki locally. I found someone who actually taught a different form of Reiki called Mahatma Reiki which is taught in three levels. I attended my first level of training in July of 2000. My sister, Marla, who lives in Ohio and had recently studied Usui Reiki herself, planned a trip to Arizona to attend the Mahatma Reiki training with me. According to my teacher, Leonie Rosenberg, "Reiki is the force behind the Yin and the Yang. It is a whole complete energy which is why the Mahatma Reiki System of Natural Healing can be used any time, any place, and under any conditions. One of the unique features of Reiki is the ease in which Reiki is learned. It is passed from a Master Teacher to a student via the 'attunement process.' During this deeply relaxing and profound experience, an energy transmission occurs and the recipient becomes able to channel divinely guided life-force energy."

During the first level of Mahatma Reiki training, participants are given opportunities to practice channeling this life force energy through their hands to others. One person lies on his or her back on a massage table while other participants in the class lay their hands on or just above the person lying on the table. The energy exchange is truly amazing whether you are the one giving Reiki or receiving Reiki. It is as though a warm energetic life force pours down from above through your body and out your hands. Typically, the hands of the person giving Reiki will become very warm. By laying your hands on the person and allowing the energy to pour through, the energy of the person on the table becomes more balanced and free flowing thus leading to needed healing within the body. Each individual has a physical, emotional, mental, and spiritual body and Reiki promotes healing as well as the integration of these bodies.

We also learned during Mahatma Reiki Level I that you can channel this life-force energy into and throughout your own body. Because of all the medications I was taking, I believed my liver was being over-taxed. I was already taking the Milk Thistle herb to help cleanse and heal my liver, but thought I could do even more. So, I would merely lay my hands over the liver area and allow the energy to flow through my hands into the liver in order to release the toxins there. I would also lay my hands on all parts of my head in order to allow healing energy to flow through and within my brain. I believe this helped all of the neurotransmitters in my brain to function more effectively.

Sometimes participants from the class would get together to participate in what is called a "Reiki Circle" or "Healing Circle." I would try to attend these gatherings as often as possible because I always felt so much better and much more highly energized after participating. In Reiki Circle, the same procedure is used as described earlier where one person lies on the table while the others stand or sit around the table and allow the divine life force energy to flow through them and onto or into the person on the table. Whether or not you believe in this type of healing, I cannot imagine anyone not feeling better after having been the person lying on the table. Most people go into a very deep, restful, meditative state and don't want to come back to full consciousness.

I believe my introduction to and continued practice of Mahatma Reiki on myself only served to strengthen my belief that the hallucinatory voices would never return. I felt I was pouring divine healing energy into my brain that would prevent any harmful or intrusive energy from residing there. Another wonderful benefit of learning a healing art such as Mahatma Reiki is that you are exposed to such warm and caring people who quite often are closely in alignment with their healing paths and missions in life. As role models, they inspired me to reflect on and clarify my own life's mission.

Mahatma Reiki also allowed me to recognize the benefits of both giving and receiving energy and how wonderful both can feel. It allowed me to remember how to look outside of myself for opportunities to give to others. I think I have always had a giving personality, but, with the onset of the schizophrenia and depression, I had turned inward. I will dare to state that I believe many people who end up developing schizophrenia, depression, or other form of mental illness in their lives are quite sensitive, get their feelings hurt easily, wear their hearts on their sleeves, and are empathic to the point where they easily feel others' pain even if only viewing someone getting hurt in a movie or on a television show. After experiencing so much hurt, sadness, and depression, it might just feel easier and safer to turn inward and not put one's feelings or self out there only to be hurt and disappointed again.

I have had to learn that, for the most part, the actions and behaviors of others are so much more about them rather than about me. To me, this means that when other seem, in my mind, to be distant, say things that hurt my feelings, or disappoint me, I need to ask myself questions such as: Is this person going through some sort of stress or trouble in their own life? Is this person's self-esteem suffering or low right now? Do I really think this person is purposely trying to hurt me? What can I do to raise my own vibration spiritually, emotionally, and mentally in order to attract vibrationally, like-minded people into my life? Or What actions can I take to reach out to the people I miss to let them know they are loved and cared for by me? The answers to these last two questions require love, time, work, and effort. An incredibly wonderful way I have found that results in my own joy, hope, happiness, and health is to find ways to give to others. One of the ways I thought I could give more to others was by volunteering at a local mental health agency in order to help and support others diagnosed with mental illness.

VOLUNTEER WORK

Because I felt I had made such significant strides in overcoming my symptoms of schizophrenia, I was incredibly grateful. I was doing so well. I decided that I should volunteer at a local mental health agency in order to try and provide support to others suffering from this illness that were not doing so well. I met with several mental health care specialists at the agency and attended several meetings before deciding on the possibility of hosting and facilitating a support group for those with schizophrenia. Although this mental health agency had a long list of support groups already in progress for the disorders of depression, manic depression, and obsessive compulsive disorder, no groups in the area were currently meeting for people with schizophrenia. I found this odd. I wanted to sit in on a few support groups for schizophrenia before I started one of my own. Since none was available, it was recommended to me that I sit in on an existing support group of individuals suffering from obsessive compulsive disorder.

Attending the group for those with obsessive compulsive disorder (as an observer) was extremely enlightening. I had no idea that there were people out there who were completely debilitated by their compulsions and unable to work because of them. After listening to their stories, I left feeling very sad for them. As an example, I remember one fellow who was in a wheelchair who talked about sitting at home all day thinking about the line where the wall and the ceiling meet and how that line was "watching" him. That is what he obsessed about all day. I believe much of the information I am presenting in this book might also be helpful to those with obsessive compulsive disorder. Learning to interrupt the thoughts you are thinking and replace them with music, positive thoughts, and positive actions might help someone with obsessive compulsive disorder break the cycle of obsession and compulsion. There are many other strategies within this book that might assist someone with this disorder in recapturing his or her mind.

The mental health agency and I decided to move forward with the idea of forming a support group for those with schizophrenia. We identified a time and location and notified doctors of this opportunity for their patients. We did other advertising as well. Our plan was to start the group in early 2001 and meet once a month on Saturday mornings. It made me feel a greater sense of purpose just knowing I was trying to help others with schizophrenia.

Also, near the end of the year 2000 and into the new year of 2001, I, for some reason, became highly motivated to clean out my condominium. I was not traveling as much for work and had a little more time at home. I had lived in my condominium for 16 years, and, even though my home was small, I had accumulated much too much "stuff." Beginning in November, I took one room a weekend and cleaned and cleared out things I did not want or need anymore. I made several donations and probably filled our dumpster three times over. But, after all the cleaning, I felt great! I really believe that when you clear out old and no longer meaningful "stuff" from your life, you make room for new and, hopefully, meaningful people, things, and experiences to come in. This is a wonderfully energizing strategy!

I would like to close this chapter by reviewing the several strategies I have presented thus far that proved helpful in my recovery from schizophrenia and depression. I believe they are strategies that can be useful to anyone wanting to improve his or her life.

STRATEGY REVIEW
1. Identify your gifts
2. Get a psychiatrist or therapist who will talk to you about your problems
3. Get appropriate medication if needed
4. Find ten things to be grateful for everyday
5. Research and gain insight into your disorder

6. Exercise daily
7. Develop a support structure including family, friends, and community
8. Find new and interesting things to learn about
9. Keep noticing gifts that come into your life
10. Identify your life's purpose
11. Participate in a healing art such as Reiki
12. Identify your process of dealing with setbacks in life
13. Take steps to lose weight (if needed) and eat healthy
14. Write down daily what you eat and plan your next day's healthy diet
15. When/if a hallucinatory "voice" intrudes or is about to intrude, replace it with singing a song in your head, thinking about a positive event or goal for the future, or remembering something positive from your past
16. Work on your self-esteem and fill yourself up with positive statements, feelings, and affirmations everyday
17. Meditate daily
18. Learn about herbs and vitamins that will benefit your health
19. Get out and volunteer
20. Find ways to give to others
21. Clean your house and donate what you no longer want or need

After reviewing these twenty-one strategies, circle the numbers of five of the strategies that you would be willing to start utilizing today. Write the five strategies you chose.

READER'S WORKBOOK: STRATEGIES YOU ARE WILLING TO TRY STARTING TODAY

1. _____

_____

2. _____

_____

3. _____

_____

4. _____

_____

5. _____

_____

CHAPTER FIVE

Learning New Strategies

E arly in 2001, I began to feel as though I had "beaten" this illness called schizophrenia. It had been over six months since I had allowed myself to hear the "voice." I wanted to share my success with others by establishing a support group for those with schizophrenia. Before the group had its first meeting, however, I decided to do more research on the disorder. I read an incredibly eye opening book by Torrey entitled *Surviving Schizophrenia*. In this text, Torrey provides current research, insights, and strategies for families, consumers (those with schizophrenia), and health care providers to use in order for those suffering with schizophrenia to live more functionally in society. It was very enlightening. I had only my own experiences with schizophrenia to inform me of what this mental illness was all about.

After reading Torrey's book, I realized that most who suffer from schizophrenia were having a much more difficult time dealing with and living with the illness than I. The book educated me regarding the prevalence of the disorder and how debilitating it can be. As I mentioned earlier in chapter two, many with schizophrenia are hospitalized and/or institutionalized for extended periods of time or even for the rest of their lives. Numerous others with schizophrenia are imprisoned, homeless, or impoverished. There are still others who cannot hold a job, but live in group homes. Some refuse to take their medications or take them erratically, thus living a nightmarish existence. Family members become dismayed, discouraged, and depressed from their attempts to provide support to the schizophrenic. It is common for those suffering from schizophrenia to not want to bathe. And, more tragically, it is common for schizophrenics to commit suicide.

From reading Torrey's book, it became clear to me that, more often than not, a person with schizophrenia will not lead a functional life. The book did not even mention that one could function without the medications altogether. Some hope was given that, if patients were consistently taking the correct medication(s), and receiving therapy, they might be somewhat functional in their life and work. As I read the book, I felt I was beginning to see the "real picture" of the life that many or most people with schizophrenia are living. And that picture was not mine. I realized I was unique. I had been able to stop the "voices."

Still, I wanted to host and facilitate the support group and help others as much as I could. We had advertised extensively with doctors and mental health agencies and I was ready to go. For four months in a row, I showed up at our agreed upon location and waited and waited. But, no one ever showed up for the support group meetings. At this point, I decided that I had tried and conceded that maybe this was not meant to be. I notified the mental health agency and we agreed to cancel the group.

During the year 2001, I met with my psychiatrist only four times. In February, he was so impressed with my success at stopping the voices that he reduced the dosage of my antipsychotic to 10mg. a day. Late in 2000, he had reduced the antidepressant to 150mg. a day. During our session in June, it was interesting that my psychiatrist advised me that the best way to function everyday was just to forget that I even had schizophrenia. After he said this, I realized that maybe it really was all for the best that my support group had not materialized. If the group had been well-attended and on-going, I may have focused too much of my thinking on the fact that I had schizophrenia. By not even having the group, I was better able to forget about the illness I once had. It was also during this session with my psychiatrist that he first recommended a book for me to read. It was by Spencer Johnson and entitled *Who Moved My Cheese?* This book revealed ideas and truths about dealing with change in your work and in your life. Although I had always believed that I had been successful in adapting to changes throughout my life, this book offered me a different perspective that allowed me to view change in a more positive light.

As a matter of fact, during this time in my life, many positive changes were occurring for me. As I mentioned in chapter four, near the end of the year 2000, I completely cleaned out my condominium. This paved the way for me to sell my condo and buy my first house in April of 2001. I also traded in my old car for a new one. I was still working fulltime as an educational consultant and part-time for the university. My finances were in good order and I was doing very well. I never thought I would be moving into my own brand new house by myself. I had always hoped I would be married. But, I did it anyway! It was nice to have so much extra room. I even converted one of my spare bedrooms into a meditation room which I think every home should have.

I also discovered a wonderful little museum/center just two miles from my new home that was an ancient petroglyph site of over 1000 petroglyphs (rock carvings in this case) on 600 boulders which were created by Native Americans including the Archaic, the Patayan, and the Hohokam Indians. I began to walk down to the museum every day for exercise. As I got to know the place and the people who worked there, I offered to volunteer once a month in leading museum tours on Saturday mornings. I enjoyed this immensely and was able to get involved further with the museum by participating in various field trips to other petroglyph and pictograph (painted rock drawings) sites throughout the state. Being affiliated with this rock art center gave me a stronger sense of community involvement since moving to my new home.

After reading *Who Moved My Cheese?* I began searching out other books that might prove inspiring to me. During my Mahatma Reiki Level I class, I remember someone mentioning the name of Doreen Virtue as an author who wrote about many topics including angels, chakras, eating in the light, and spiritual solutions to problems. Doreen is a psychologist who conducts angel therapy and spiritual healing. I read several of her books that summer and even had the good fortune of attending one of her workshops when she was in town. She can see your spirit guides as well as those who have passed over to the other side but are still close to you. Reading Doreen's books and seeing her in person motivated me to take a closer look at my own spirituality and look for ways to develop it further. In Doreen's books, she teaches you techniques to receive your own divine guidance. She also provides many effective meditation techniques to assist you in receiving this guidance. I have listed numerous Doreen Virtue books that I have personally read in the references.

I think because I have always intuitively known that I can access and listen to my own spiritual guidance directly from God, I was never one who believed very much in organized religion. However, I had been a member of the Bahai Faith for fifteen years of my life from age 20 to 35. As discussed earlier, my brother, Steve, introduced me to the Bahai Faith and became a Bahai before I did. I became a Bahai because I believed in several of the faith's tenets including: 1) honoring and accepting the nine major religions of the world and their believers, 2) striving to create a world that is one country, thus dissolving national boundaries and dramatically reducing the need for war, 3) acknowledging the equality of men and women throughout the world, 4) establishing a universal language that everyone in the world can use – possibly sign language, and 5) providing universal education for all. Another reason I became a Bahai was because I enjoyed the overall more positive vibration of the people I interacted with who were Bahais. I left the faith at age 35 because my experiences with the Bahai Faith left me believing that it was necessary to "convert" others to the faith to increase our numbers and feeling pressured to donate more and more money to various Bahai causes. The Bahai Faith, from my perspective, was becoming somewhat judgmental and money driven. However, the reader may wish to research further the Bahai Faith which has its beginnings in Persia (now Iran).

As I mentioned, I have always felt connected to God. I do not believe there is a single God, but, rather, believe that God is within us, around us, and everywhere. I think of God more as a force of light and love as described in Virtue's books.

I began reading other books about spirituality and health such as Wayne Dyer's *10 Secrets for Success and Inner Peace*. Some of those secrets that he elaborates on in his book include: "1) Have a mind that is open to everything and attached to nothing, 2) Embrace silence, 3) Give up your personal history, 4) Treat yourself as if you already are what you would like to be, 5) Treasure your divinity, and 6) Wisdom is avoiding all thoughts that weaken you." For someone with schizophrenia, depression, or any mental illness, number six is especially poignant. Later, I read several other Wayne Dyer books which I have listed in the references as well.

Another book I read that had a profound effect on me was Andrew Weil's *8 Weeks to Optimum Health*. In this book, Dr. Weil explains how to: "1) Build a lifestyle that protects you from premature illness and disability, 2) Improve your current eating habits so that your diet is more nutritious, 3) Incorporate basic breathing exercises into your life for greater relaxation and energy, and 4) Make art, music, and the natural world more important parts of your life." Dr. Weil provides healing testimonials from those who have made these recommended changes in their lives as well as customized plans for various age groups, men, women, groups with certain health problems, and much, much more.

A colleague of Andrew Weil's at the University of Arizona was Lewis Mehl-Madrona who I had the good fortune to attend one of his lectures. I read Dr. Mehl-Madrona's book entitled *Coyote Medicine* in which he presents a model of healing that is holistic, humanistic, and drawn from his Native American heritage. As a graduate of Stanford Medical School, Dr. Mehl-Madrona entered the world of modern medicine where he encountered doctors performing unnecessary, rushed, and even botched medical procedures. After losing his faith in conventional medicine, Mehl-Madrona turned to alternative paths to recovery and health which included attention to spiritual health. He prescribes methods of healing that integrate elements of ancient Native American rituals and religious ceremonies with modern psychology and medicine. Dr. Lewis Mehl-Madrona previously worked with Dr. Andrew Weil at the University of Arizona's Program for Integrative Medicine in Tucson, Arizona.

A final book that I will discuss in this chapter that had a huge impact on me was Dr. Phil McGraw's *Self Matters*. I believe this book was so important because it motivated me to take a good look at my authentic self which, according to Dr. Phil, is "that person you once were before life took its toll. It is the person you have always wanted to be, but were too distracted, busy, or scared to become." In reading his and the other books previously mentioned, the insight came to me that, in order to find my authentic self, I would need to peel off the layer of the medications which, to a certain extent, deadened me. I wasn't sure how I would do this successfully, but the seed was planted.

Now, it is the reader's turn to identify several books, authors, lectures, or workshops that have had an impact on your life or inspired you to move in a new and improved direction in your life:

READER'S WORKBOOK: INSPIRED LEARNINGS

New Learning #1:

_____

_____

_____

_____

_____

_____

_____

_____

_____

_____

_____

_____

Source: (Book, Author, Lecture, Workshop, Etc.)

_____

_____

_____

_____

_____

_____

_____

_____

_____

_____

_____

_____

_____

_____

_____

_____

How has this new learning improved your life?

_____

_____

_____

_____

_____

_____

_____

_____

_____

_____

_____

_____

_____

_____

_____

New Learning #2:

_____

_____

_____

_____

_____

_____

_____

_____

_____

_____

_____

_____

_____

_____

_____

_____

Source: (Book, Author, Lecture, Workshop, Etc.)

_____

_____

_____

_____

_____

_____

_____

_____

_____

_____

_____

_____

_____

_____

How has this new learning improved your life?

_____

_____

_____

_____

_____

_____

_____

_____

_____

_____

_____

_____

_____

_____

_____

_____

New Learning #3:

_____

_____

_____

_____

_____

_____

_____

_____

_____

_____

_____

_____

_____

_____

_____

_____

Source: (Book, Author, Lecture, Workshop, Etc.)

_____

_____

_____

_____

_____

_____

_____

_____

_____

_____

_____

_____

_____

_____

_____

How has this new learning improved your life?

New Learning #4:

_____

_____

_____

_____

_____

_____

_____

_____

_____

_____

_____

_____

_____

_____

_____

Source: (Book, Author, Lecture, Workshop, Etc.)

_____

_____

_____

_____

_____

_____

_____

_____

_____

_____

_____

_____

_____

_____

_____

_____

How has this new learning improved your life?

_____

_____

_____

_____

_____

_____

_____

_____

_____

_____

_____

_____

_____

_____

_____

New Learning #5:

Source: (Book, Author, Lecture, Workshop, Etc.)

_____

_____

_____

_____

_____

_____

_____

_____

_____

_____

_____

_____

_____

_____

_____

How has this new learning improved your life?

For me, the year 2001 was a year of incredible learning and opening up to new possibilities personally, emotionally, intellectually, spiritually, and physically. Good things were happening in my workplace as well. I began to do more traveling for my company as they had asked me to undertake training to become an educational curriculum auditor where I would learn to audit schools and districts that were potential or current customers with the purpose of identifying areas where our company could provide services. This was challenging yet exciting. The three levels of audit training took me to San Diego for Level I in January, Seattle for Level II in May, and Tucson for Level III in December. The work was stimulating, interesting, and in alignment with my purpose of helping children receive a quality education.

As you have seen throughout this book, I like to take time to identify the many gifts that have been given to me that have made my life better. This strategy of being in gratitude always infuses me with hope and promise for the future. In 2001, I was grateful for:

MORE GIFTS

1. Getting to visit with my brother, Steve, in San Diego
2. Reduction in dosages of medications
3. Reading many books that offered me new and different perspectives
4. Buying a new house and new car
5. Volunteering at the rock art center
6. Curriculum audit training

Within this chapter, I have shared some of my personal spiritual beliefs along with one of my life's purposes which is to support others suffering from schizophrenia or mental illness. As this chapter closes, it is now your turn. Take Dr. Phil's advice and reflect on that person you once were before life took its toll on you. Who have you always wanted to be, but were too distracted, busy, or scared to become? Then think about those spiritual beliefs you possess that represent and support who you really are – your authentic self. For this assignment, there will be three parts. First, write about who you think your authentic self really is. You may not know completely, but give it a try and go with your gut feelings. Second, write about your true spiritual beliefs. Do not write about the beliefs that have been imposed upon you in childhood and over the years. Tell what you truly believe about your own spirituality. Last, describe what your life's purpose is. You may have several. I know I do.

READER'S WORKBOOK: DESCRIBE YOUR AUTHENTIC SELF

Who is this person you have always wanted to be?

_____

_____

_____

_____

_____

_____

_____

_____

_____

_____

_____

_____

_____

DESCRIBE YOUR PERSONAL SPIRITUAL BELIEFS

What are your true spiritual beliefs?

_____

_____

_____

_____

_____

_____

_____

_____

_____

_____

_____

_____

_____

_____

YOUR LIFE'S PURPOSE

What is your purpose or mission in life?

_____

_____

_____

_____

_____

_____

_____

_____

_____

_____

_____

_____

_____

_____

CHAPTER SIX

A Major Setback and a Miracle

Early in 2002, my psychiatrist continued to lower my medication dosages. My body seemed to be adjusting very well to the lower dosages. I felt more energy and didn't need as much sleep. I was maintaining my Weight Watchers goal weight of 110 pounds. All was going very well in my educational consulting position. Late in January, I was scheduled to present several in-services for an inner-city school district in Ohio which happened to be located not far from Dayton, Ohio, the town in which I grew up. I had two brothers and a sister still living there, so I made arrangements to visit them for a few days after my in-service trainings were completed. This would be the last time I would see my brother, Steve, physically alive on planet Earth. While in Dayton, I stayed with my sister, Marla. One night, my brother, Steve, invited us to his house along with my brother, David, and my nephew, Trevor (David's son), who both live in Dayton as well. While at Steve's, we all took a tour of his new home into which he had recently moved. I could tell how proud Steve was to be renting a house rather than an apartment. He gave us the royal tour! My niece, Michelle, and her then boyfriend, Chris, came over to Steve's house, too, for the get together. We had a great time enjoying each other's company and eating our favorite hometown Joe's Pizza. I really could not tell that anything was wrong with Steve although I did notice that he was continuing to struggle with being overweight.

At the end of the evening, we all hugged and said our goodbyes. Steve told me he would pick me up in the morning from my sister, Marla's place and drive me to the airport in Columbus, Ohio. The next morning, Steve called early. I happened to answer the phone at my sister's. Steve let me know that he could not take me to the airport after all because he had awakened with a severe migraine headache and was too ill to drive. He asked if my sister would take me to the airport. I talked with Steve a few minutes more and I remember telling him that I hoped he felt better soon. As we hung up, I had this sinking feeling in the pit of my stomach that told me I would never talk with or see Steve again.

In February, I was asked to serve on an audit team which would be responsible for auditing a large inner-city school district in the Northeast. The district was comprised of over 180 schools. A large team of over 25 auditors was assembled for the task. I served as an intern since this was my first audit experience. I had the fortunate opportunity to meet and collaborate with education professionals from all across the United States. Even though it was very difficult work, I enjoyed the audit experience immensely. I felt a strong sense of fulfilling one of my missions or purposes in life by working to help this school district which was "in trouble."

I continued with my volunteer work at the rock art center by leading Saturday morning tours. My life seemed to be going very well at this point. I felt happy, more energized, and intellectually stimulated. I was regularly meditating and daily practicing yoga. I was also taking more time to get back up to our family cabin for hiking and enjoying nature. I remember one hike, in particular, that I went on during a Friday morning late in March. I had taken the day off. It was a perfectly gorgeous Arizona day just right for a long hike in the mountains. As I hiked, I remember feeling as though my mind was clear and I did not have a care in the world. After my hike, I decided to go home, get cleaned up, and meditate before going to pick up my new eyeglasses and meet my mother for dinner.

The meditation I chose for this day was one where I listened to a recording of a guided meditation. The recording guides you to relax from head to toe, breathe deeply, and imagine your spirit guides and angels communicating with you. I have practiced this particular meditation many times, and, at the end of the meditation, I could always sense the presence of my Grandmother Abbott who has passed over and a Native American guide. I could "see" them in my mind's eye with my grandmother to my right and the Native American guide to my left. My eyes, of course, were closed, but I would feel their presence every time. That day, however, at the end of the meditation, it seemed as though my meditation room was "filled" with other presences as well. Again, in my mind's eye, I could clearly see my cousin, Jimmy, who had passed over in 1989 from a car accident where he had been killed. He was in his early twenties when he died. He was near my feet as I was lying down for this meditation. Next, to my right, closer to my leg, I saw my Uncle Bill who had passed over a few years previously from cancer. He had been in his seventies when he died. Then, to my left, near my leg I was making out a presence that seemed to be more ghostly, fluid, and not as solid. My first impression was that it was my brother, Steve. But, then, I thought to myself, "This could not be. Steve is alive."

I went to pick up my eyeglasses and then join my mother at our little "meeting place" at a local mall in Scottsdale before going to dinner. One look at her face immediately told me that something was terribly wrong. She communicated to me that my brother, Steve, the one I had "seen" in my meditation room, had been shot and killed. I was completely and utterly stunned and shocked. He had always been my favorite brother and the one I had always been closest to. Steve had already passed over when he came to me in my meditation room even though I had not yet known of his death. But, because he had come to me, I had this profound sense that he was alright and at peace. It was a huge gift to me.

By the next day, we had learned that my brother had shot himself in the chest area. As I mentioned earlier, this brother had lived in San Diego. There, he ran an office cleaning business from 1982-1997. Steve loved San Diego. However, during the recession of the mid-1990s, his business began to fail. In 1997, he returned to our hometown of Dayton, Ohio, to run his own business of nursing arts in partnership with my oldest brother, Frankie. When Steve originally told me that he was planning to move from San Diego to Dayton to start a business with my brother, I intuitively and strongly felt that this was a bad idea, I told Steve so, but tried to be supportive of this new venture. After Steve moved to Dayton, Frankie ended up backing out of the partnership and let Steve know that he and his wife and children were moving out of state. Frankie left Steve to start, build, operate, and run the business on his own which Steve did from 1998 until 2002. He had 60 employees who worked with patients in their homes dispensing medications, giving baths, and all sorts of other nursing activities. My brother had apparently been having some major financial problems and, for the first time, was unable to make payroll for his employees meaning he did not have the money in the bank to pay them on that Friday. So, I think, in order to avoid the embarrassment and his employees' disappointment, he took his own life. It was a tragedy. If only he had asked for some help, things might have turned out differently. But, he had not. We, as family, had no idea that he was in such financial trouble. My brother had other troubles as well. He was overweight, not in good health, single and many times lonely, and, I believe he did not feel he had much to live for. I think he may have missed the positive energies he so loved while living in beautiful San Diego. And, in retrospect, I believe Steve might have even been suffering from the mental illness of depression.

The weeks and months that followed were very sad for me. Even though I felt extremely depressed and grief stricken, I did not feel I needed more antidepressant medication. Something inside me just "knew" that I had to go through the grief. But, there was also a part of me that felt as if it had left along with my favorite brother and a part of me wanted to go and be with him. Looking back, I am not sure exactly how I got through this time in my life. Although I did have plenty of family and friends as support, I believe I had a great deal of angelic support, too. I felt angels and spirit guides around me all of the time as I do to this day. My brother on the other side also "visits" me once in a while and is doing well. Steve still has his wonderful sense of humor, beams a powerful loving energy, and is free of his weight.

As I continued to work through my grief, I increased my efforts to get together with Reiki practitioners to help heal each other. I had continued to do Reiki on myself, but it was comforting and supportive to spend time with others who practiced Reiki. I also spent a good deal of time with my mother trying to help her get through her grief. She was completely devastated by my brother's (her son's) death as any parent of their own child would be.

When I visited my psychiatrist in May, I was remaining stable on the lower dosages of medications. He recommended other books for me to read including Brinkman and Kirschner's *Dealing with People You Can't Stand* and *Dealing with Relatives*, Rohm's *Positive Personality Profiles* and *Who Do You Think You Are Anyway?* and Kiyosaki's *Rich Dad, Poor Dad* and *Cash Flow Quadrant*. How I wished my brother could have read the Kiyosaki books, especially. They were very educational and helped me improve my own finances even further. As a result of reading Kiyosaki's two books, I stepped up my efforts to increase my savings and better plan for retirement. Also, during May, it helped me tremendously to make a list of a number of projects I had been meaning to get around to such as deep cleaning my house and the cabin. I also cleaned out and reorganized all of my files and closets. I think this was therapeutic for me in helping me work through my grief.

Back in chapter four, I reviewed several strategies that I had used to help me cope with my schizophrenia and depression. Upon reflection, I recognize that I continued to use most of these strategies to help me cope with the loss of my brother. I made a special appointment with my psychiatrist to talk about Steve's death. I even met with a counselor several times to work through my feelings of grief. I exercised daily and I continued to develop and rely upon my support structure of family, friends, and community. I participated in new learning as I completed my Mahatma Reiki Level II class in July which my sister, Marla, from Ohio came to attend as well. I continued to eat healthy and monitor my weight. I meditated daily. I continued my volunteer work at the rock art center. And, as I mentioned, I cleaned my house and worked on household projects.

But, the strategy that was most helpful of all was continuing to notice the gifts that came into my life. I came to a point late in the summer of 2002 when I was able to recognize my brother's death as a gift to me. The gift was the realization that this physical life on planet Earth is not all there is. After our physical death, we live on and have other work to do. However, while on this planet, we need to do the best we can with our lives. While my brother made the choice to end his physical existence, I knew he was still around providing me and others with support. Even when my brother was physically alive, he always encouraged me to do my best. I regret that I did not encourage him more to do the same.

So, out of this loss emerged a better me – one that now had a much stronger commitment to doing this physical life better. I became clearer regarding my mission in life. I worked harder to maintain a high self-esteem. I looked for reasons to be hopeful and helpful. I also wanted to feel more of my inner spirit come alive. One way I thought I could achieve this was by getting off of my antipsychotic and antidepressant medications completely. Granted, I was on much lower dosages at this point. But, my new goal was to live successfully and happily without them.

In November of 2002, part of my wish was granted. At this time, surprisingly, it was my psychiatrist who recommended that I discontinue the antipsychotic medication altogether. It had been over two years since I had allowed the "voice" to intrude on my mind. I had no other symptoms associated with schizophrenia. I continued to take the antidepressant medication as my psychiatrist explained I needed to remain on it for at least another year while I stabilized and adjusted to being off of the antipsychotic. I experienced withdrawal symptoms from going off of the antipsychotic including insomnia and headaches. It felt as though a heavy cloud was being lifted from my brain. But, I was determined. The withdrawal symptoms lasted for a little over one month and I continued to exercise, meditate, eat healthy, and think positively. As 2002 ended, I was, miraculously, completely off of the antipsychotic medication!

A final wonderful ending to 2002 occurred because of a conversation I had with the counselor I had seen soon after my brother had passed. As mentioned earlier, I met with this counselor for several sessions to help me deal with the grief of the loss. I shared with her the idea that I wish I could have had the chance to say goodbye to my brother, Steve. She recommended I see an acquaintance of hers who is a clairvoyant and psychic consultant who also does medium work which involves contacting those on the other side who have passed over. I made an appointment to see this "medium" over the Christmas holiday season since my sister, Marla, would be in town from Ohio to visit and we would be able to meet with the medium and, hopefully, have communication with Steve. He was so important to both of us. Our medium tuned right in to our brother and how he had passed describing the scene exactly without any help from us. We were told that he is doing well and that he loves us both. We learned that he is often around us and his nieces, nephews, brother, father, and mother. The medium mentioned specific times when he had visited us recently. He had been right behind me while I was working on my computer at work and I had felt his presence back at that time. My sister and I were both very impressed by the medium's accuracy and we left feeling as though we connected with our brother and there was a huge amount of love between us all. Even today, every time I see a hawk overhead, I feel it is my brother, Steve, stopping by to say hello, to lend an ear, and oftentimes to give advice. When I ask him a question, I can hear his answer loud and clear in my head. I, myself, have experienced my ability to connect with the other side just as I had when my brother first crossed over before I even knew on this plane that he had physically passed. I also believe that a great many people have this gift of connecting with the other side and being "visited" here on this physical plane by loved ones who have passed on. The name of the psychic medium that connected with our brother is Carrie Shubert and she lives in Scottsdale, Arizona. I have listed one of her books and one of her CDs in the references and recommended reading section at the end of this book.

Before moving on to the next chapter, I would like to give you, the reader, an opportunity to think about how you can "do" or "experience" this physical life on planet Earth better. This will be a goal-setting session. Review all facets of your life and identify how you can grow in each. You may be neglecting certain areas of your life more than others. The first step is to list some ideas of how you would like to do better in the following specific areas of your life:

READER'S WORKBOOK: FACETS OF LIFE GOAL-SETTING

1. Personal Self-Esteem

I would like to improve in this area by doing the following:

_____

_____

_____

_____

_____

_____

_____

_____

_____

_____

_____

_____

_____

_____

2. Family Relationships

I would like to improve in this area by doing the following:

_____

_____

_____

_____

_____

_____

_____

_____

_____

_____

_____

_____

_____

3. Relationships with Friends

I would like to improve in this area by doing the following:

_____

_____

_____

_____

_____

_____

_____

_____

_____

_____

_____

_____

_____

4. Romantic Relationships

I would like to improve in this area by doing the following:

_____

_____

_____

_____

_____

_____

_____

_____

_____

_____

_____

_____

_____

_____

_____

5. Personal Health

I would like to improve in this area by doing the following:

_____

_____

_____

_____

_____

_____

_____

_____

_____

_____

_____

_____

_____

_____

6. Body Image

I would like to improve in this area by doing the following:

_____

_____

_____

_____

_____

_____

_____

_____

_____

_____

_____

_____

_____

_____

_____

7. Work/Career

I would like to improve in this area by doing the following:

_____

_____

_____

_____

_____

_____

_____

_____

_____

_____

_____

_____

_____

_____

8. Personal Finances

I would like to improve in this area by doing the following:

_____

_____

_____

_____

_____

_____

_____

_____

_____

_____

_____

_____

_____

_____

_____

9. Continuing Education

I would like to improve in this area by doing the following:

_____

_____

_____

_____

_____

_____

_____

_____

_____

_____

_____

_____

_____

_____

_____

10. Spiritual Growth

I would like to improve in this area by doing the following:

_____

_____

_____

_____

_____

_____

_____

_____

_____

_____

_____

_____

_____

_____

11. Service to the Planet

I would like to improve in this area by doing the following:

_____

_____

_____

_____

_____

_____

_____

_____

_____

_____

_____

_____

_____

12. Expressing Creativity

I would like to improve in this area by doing the following:

_____

_____

_____

_____

_____

_____

_____

_____

_____

_____

_____

_____

_____

_____

13. Other:

I would like to improve in this area by doing the following:

Choose only two or three of the areas to focus on and begin to make plans to implement some of your ideas in order to improve your life. The mere act of thinking about these areas and writing down your ideas for improvement sets in motion their accomplishment. Later in this book I will describe a process for the reader to use to turn goals into achievements using a strategy that incorporates the use of positive affirmations.

CHAPTER SEVEN

Complete Recovery From Schizophrenia and Depression

As I moved forward into the year 2003, I felt that my mind, body, and spirit were all adjusting well to being without the antipsychotic medication that I had been taking since 1998. I was finally in a place where I wanted to reach out and find someone to date or have a relationship with. I had not been out on a date since 1996. I began attending a local new-age type church where I met several very nice gentlemen. I attended a class with one and even went out on a date with him, but we really didn't "click." However, I was very proud of myself that I took this first step.

Just as I began to feel that I might be able to have a social life with men again, my company began sending me "on the road" to do in-services for several weeks out of each month. I traveled to California, Alabama, Illinois, Louisiana, North Carolina, Texas, Ohio, and New York. It was difficult to establish or maintain a social life with all of the traveling. It seemed I only had time to do laundry and repack between trips. Even though I was asked to travel extensively, the company I was working for was losing business and downsizing dramatically. Within approximately one year's time, the company trimmed down from 120 employees to 60. I began to worry about the future of the company and my future there as well. It seemed that the 60 employees were being asked to do the work of 90. I was so busy with my fulltime work that I decided it would be best to end my part-time work at the local university for which I had taught graduate level distance learning classes for the past four years.

I clearly recall the moment when I decided that I had had enough of all the traveling and needed to look for fulltime employment elsewhere. I was just returning from a four day trip to an elementary school in inner city New York. The in-services I had presented were held on a Friday and a Saturday for teachers and administrators. My flight from New York City to Phoenix was on Sunday, but had been delayed. I already had another bag packed at home and ready to go because I was scheduled to leave early Monday morning (the next day) for LAX to work with several high schools in inner city Los Angeles. I was flying on the same airline for both trips. When I arrived in Phoenix from New York City, it was about 10:00pm. As I came through the gate, I looked up at the monitor that lists the upcoming flight departures. The flight I was to leave on the next morning at 7:00am was already listed on the monitor. What a depressing moment! I did complain to my supervisor at work, and, primarily because the need for in-services was declining due to reduced sales, my travel schedule slowed down by June.

It was at about this time that I began to update my resume and pursue work that might not involve so much travel and look again into teaching fulltime at the university level. For the most part, I had been happy working as an educational consultant for the company, but I was very worried about their future. From February to July of 2003, another 15 employees were laid off. I felt it might only be a matter of time before I was let go as well. So, I decided to be proactive and find something else soon. After applying to and participating in a number of interviews, I was hired by Northern Arizona University to teach undergraduate elementary education courses to cohorts (groups) of students in the Phoenix area. The job offer was made to me in November and I started work in December, 2003. I was very excited to begin teaching at the university level fulltime.

Earlier in about June or July of 2003, I happened upon a group of people who met once or twice a month just to meditate together. I was still hoping to find a nice, spiritual guy to date, so I thought this might be a possible place to meet someone. I also wanted to meet new friends. The couple who held the meditation group at their home was warm and welcoming. They were also involved in healing arts such as acupuncture and grief counseling. Whenever I attended, I left feeling more healed. I think we sometimes make the mistake of thinking we only need to heal physically. But, I believe we need continual healing of our emotions, our minds, our spirits, and our physical bodies. Attending this meditation group helped me to become more in tune with the other areas of my life that needed healing.

It was also during this time, during the second half of 2003, that I began to notice how strong my intuitions and psychic impressions were. My intuition and sixth sense became more pronounced and on target. Rather than rely on my logic as I had always done in the past, I started to go with my intuition in making decisions about where to go in my life. I believe everyone has this ability and it has a great deal to do with being your "authentic self" as Dr. Phil described it. Living according to my intuition and sixth sense contributed to an increased faith in myself and trust in the universe. I was beginning to live much more in harmony with the world rather than in fear of it.

During much of 2003, I began to think about how I could contribute to the world and help protect its environment. At the one year anniversary of the passing of my brother, Steve, I decided to plant his favorite tree (mesquite) in his honor behind our family cabin. This small act had a strong healing effect and allowed me to release more of the grief I felt because of his death. This may sound strange, but, since my brother's death, I have felt as though he visits and communicates with me more than ever. It has been extremely comforting to know he is around and to know he is doing well.

Another way I thought I could help protect our planet and environment was to become a site steward in Arizona. This is someone who undergoes training and is assigned one or more archaeological sites in the state to visit periodically in order to ensure that the sites are not being defaced or damaged, thus, protecting our Native American heritage. Since I love to hike, I thought this would be a perfect activity for me. I also thought this would be a good way to meet some like-minded people. In November of 2003, I participated in the two day training and, in December, was assigned my two sites in a nearby wilderness area.

During my visit with my psychiatrist in November of 2003, we both celebrated the fact that I had been completely off of the antipsychotic medication for a full year. At one point earlier in my therapy, my psychiatrist had informed me that if a patient is able to live without the medication and without the symptoms of schizophrenia for two years, then he or she no longer has to retain the diagnosis of schizophrenia. I should remind the reader that very few individuals are able to accomplish these two things (no medication and no symptoms). But, at this point, I was certain I would be one who could and would. My primary purpose for writing this book is to share with others how I did it and offer inspiration, suggestions, and strategies for how someone diagnosed with schizophrenia might be able to move toward and, hopefully, accomplish this goal in his or her life.

It was now time to withdraw from the low dosage of the antidepressant. My psychiatrist believed I was ready to do this. I thought I was ready to clear this final hurdle as well. But, I almost did not achieve it. Withdrawing from the antidepressant, for me, was even more difficult than withdrawing from the antipsychotic. The insomnia was worse and it was extremely hard for me to focus my vision. If I turned my head suddenly to look at something, it was as though my brain was "shivering" and had to work extremely hard to "catch up" to the new object or view. I was unable to stay off of the medication during the first month I tried. When I returned to see my psychiatrist in December, I reported that the withdrawal symptoms were so severe that I had to resume taking the medication. When he explained that I might have to stay on the medication for the rest of my life, I decided to give it another try. Several times during December, I almost resumed taking the medication, but I would talk myself out of it by thinking, "A month from now you will feel so much better if you just stick it out." I suffered incredibly painful headaches as well.

I made the mistake of going online to see how successful others had been at withdrawing from this medication. I read one nightmare after another about how unsuccessful others had been. Some became suicidal while others landed in the hospital. You might want to try looking up this information for yourself sometime. I think you will, at the very least, be horrified at what you learn about the difficulty of getting off of antidepressant drugs. It was two full months before I felt better, but I actually did accomplish getting off of this medication (Applause please!!).

I don't mean to criticize the use of antidepressant medication. For several years, I needed it to function and to not feel depressed. The antidepressant I took works to increase the level of serotonin in the brain which makes you feel better. After going off of the antidepressant, I had to work harder than ever on a daily basis to keep my spirits and self-esteem high. But, at this point, I had developed the tools and strategies necessary to do just that. It has been a long process of incorporating these tools and strategies into habits of living. And, that is the key. They must become lifestyle habits. It might be easier to take the pills. But, for me, my life was just not as fulfilling as I thought it could or should be. The hard work of developing positive and healthy lifestyle habits feels good to me and I hope it feels good or will feel good to you as well.

Before I continue with the final two chapters of this book where I talk about what I have done to establish and maintain a well-balanced life free of schizophrenia and depression from 2004 to the present (2012), it is time for me to share the many gifts that emerged in my life from 2000-2003. After my list of additional gifts, there is a Reader's Workbook in which the reader can write additional personal gifts that might have come to mind since listing your original gifts back in chapter one. If you are a family member, friend, or caregiver of one who is mentally ill, perhaps you could instead list the gifts you see in your loved one or the one you care for and explain why or how each has been or continues to be a gift in his or her and your own life.

MORE GIFTS

1. Continuing on Weight Watchers
2. Learning to maintain a high self-esteem
3. Mahatma Reiki
4. Visit with psychic medium, Carrie Shubert
5. Healing from my brother, Steve's, passing
6. Still more books
7. Meditation group
8. New job as a university professor
9. Becoming a site steward
10. Withdrawal from antipsychotic and antidepressant medications

READER'S WORKBOOK: MORE OF YOUR GIFTS

1. _____

Why or how has this been a gift?

_____

_____

_____

_____

_____

_____

_____

2. _____

Why or how has this been a gift?

_____

_____

_____

_____

_____

_____

_____

3. _____

Why or how has this been a gift?

_____

_____

_____

_____

_____

_____

_____

4. _____

Why or how has this been a gift?

_____

_____

_____

_____

_____

_____

_____

5. _____

Why or how has this been a gift?

_____

_____

_____

_____

_____

_____

_____

6. _____

Why or how has this been a gift?

_____

_____

_____

_____

_____

_____

_____

7. _____

Why or how has this been a gift?

_____

_____

_____

_____

_____

_____

_____

8. _____

Why or how has this been a gift?

_____

_____

_____

_____

_____

_____

_____

9. _____

Why or how has this been a gift?

_____

_____

_____

_____

_____

_____

10. _____

Why or how has this been a gift?

_____

_____

_____

_____

_____

_____

CHAPTER EIGHT

Understanding What Happened and Creating a Well Balanced Life

The year 2004 was one of wonderful opportunities in many areas of my life including intellectually, academically, physically, psychologically, and spiritually. My new job as a university professor was and continues to be exciting and interesting. I spent much of spring, 2004, preparing for the classes I would be teaching in the fall. I felt aligned with my purpose of helping pre-service teachers prepare to become fulltime elementary school teachers. The enthusiasm my undergraduate students displayed and continue to display is inspiring. I have taught and continue to teach classes on School and Society, Literacy, Curriculum, Assessment, and Classroom Management. It has been intellectually stimulating for me to prepare these courses for my students. I also continued with my training in curriculum auditing by attending seminars in Florida and Montana throughout the year. I shared some of my training with fellow university professors in the spring of 2004.

I have continued to work on myself physically to stay fit and heal my body. All of the medications I had previously taken needed to be cleansed from my body. The liver has had to work hard for many years to process all of the aspirin, antihistamines, nasal sprays, antidepressants, and antipsychotics I had taken. I needed to rejuvenate my body and all of its organs in order to allow my life force to efficiently flow. I have reduced my consumption of soda pop. I eat very little meat because meat is dead and has no life force. I read a book by Doreen Virtue entitled *Eating in the Light* which transformed my way of thinking about food and drink. I make concerted efforts to infuse my body with food that has greater life force in it such as fruits, vegetables, nuts, and grains. I also take daily vitamin and nutritional supplements.

I read a book by Yogi Ramacharaka called *The Hindu Yogi Practical Water Cure* which was written back in 1909. In it he explains how we can aerate or infuse the water we drink with more prana or life force just by pouring it from glass to glass or pitcher to glass infusing the water with bubbles of air and life force before we drink it. I've also made it a habit to bless my food and water before ingesting them. This allows the food/water to fill me with more life and energy.

In February, 2004, I attended a sweat lodge with a highly regarded and reputable shaman to further cleanse my body of toxins. It was a wonderful healing experience. I breathed in all of the hot steam created in the lodge due to water being poured on hot stones. For several days afterward, I felt as though I was coughing up toxins from deep in my lungs. I had lived with one or more cigarette smokers in the house from birth to age 23, and I believe there was still residue in my lungs that needed to be cleaned out.

In March of 2004, I visited my psychiatrist for the last time. He explained that I was doing extremely well and did not need to come back to see him unless, at some point in the future, I felt I needed to. It was at this point I celebrated the fact that I was leaving the entire four to five year episode of my schizophrenia and depression behind me. I was physically and mentally healed and wanted to create a positive future for myself. To begin this process, I signed up for a class that was offered at a local, new age bookstore called "Creating Your Heart's Desire." The class was based on the book by Sonia Choquette entitled *Your Heart's Desire*. The class met for four months and it involved a good deal of self-reflection on areas in my life where I desired to manifest new and better creations. The area I focused on was relationships. I desired better relationships with family and friends and wished to create a new romantic relationship with just the right person for me. Before I could create this new romantic relationship, however, I realized that I still needed to heal myself emotionally of several past relationships.

Fortunately, I was somehow guided to just the right person to help me do this. She is a healer who does energy work with people to help them release old wounds, honor their inner child, retrieve soul fragments, and develop into "Lightbodies" here on planet Earth so that we, together, can raise the vibration and consciousness of the planet. An excellent book on this subject is *What is Lightbody?* by Taichi-ren and is listed in the references and recommended reading section at the end of this book. Over the summer of 2004, I had several treatments with this healer and was able to release most of the remaining grief over the death of my brother as well as hurts and fears I had held from past romantic relationships. This healer also assisted me in clarifying my life mission and has inspired and supported me in thinking about writing this book to help others.

Additionally, this healer taught me a strategy to mentally raise the level of serotonin in my brain. She asked me to meditate and go to my brain and intuitively ascertain its current level of serotonin. It can be thought of as a thermometer from zero to one hundred. When I "tune in" to the level, I usually get a measure of sixty to sixty-five. But, then, she taught me to mentally imagine the level increasing to a higher number that feels good. I usually mentally raise the serotonin level to eighty or eighty-five. This has been very helpful to me. She also asked me to "tune in" to that serotonin level every day to see where it is. For me, some days when I tune in, it is at sixty while other days it may be at seventy or seventy-five. I practice this every day, and, while it may just be my imagination, I actually do feel better and more positive.

I truly believe, however, that our physical, emotional, mental, and spiritual healing is never complete. It is a life-long process that involves the uncovering of who we really are and what we are meant to do and be in our quest to become more whole. A book that has helped me tremendously in understanding this idea is by Helen Schucman entitled *A Course in Miracles*. This is a book that is read over the course of a year and involves the practice of daily lessons. Many people have taken this course including Wayne Dyer, Doreen Virtue, and Marianne Williamson. (I have already listed in the references and recommended reading section at the end of this book those books by Wayne Dyer and Doreen Virtue that have positively affected me. I also read the wonderful book by Marianne Williamson entitled *Everyday Grace* and have listed it in the references as well.) A basic premise of *A Course in Miracles* is that "The world we see merely reflects our own internal frame of reference and that, as we change our thinking about the world, we change the world we see." Again, this is a daily process. I joined a study group at the local Unity Church in order to more fully apply these ideas in my life. I have learned so much about how my own thoughts can affect me, my body, my world, and others.

Dr. Masaru Emoto, in his book *The Hidden Messages in Water*, presents his decade long research on the effects of thoughts and words on the crystal formations in water. In his study, Dr. Emoto has found that water from clear springs and water that has been exposed to loving words show brilliant, complex, colorful, and crisp snowflake patterns of crystals while polluted water or water exposed to negative thoughts, forms incomplete, asymmetrical, and oily patterns with dull colors. And, because the human body mostly consists of water, Dr. Emoto believes our thoughts can have a profound impact on ourselves.

Water can also be used to clean and clear away negative thoughts and energies that a person accumulates or encounters in his or her daily life. Other basic earth elements such as lightning, fire, wind, and earth can also be utilized to clear away negative energy as I will allude to next.

RAVEN CLAN CLEARING

The healer I mentioned earlier in this chapter who was so instrumental in activating my "lightbody" and in teaching me wonderful self-healing techniques had also become a friend. Her name is Rahne (pronounced "rain"). In April, 2005, I invited Rahne to visit our family cabin north of town just to see it and to go for a little hike. This healer is also an empath and can "feel" energies that most of us are unaware of. As we entered the cabin, I could tell she was "feeling" something out of the ordinary. I invited her to see the two upstairs rooms, but, when we entered the large bedroom upstairs, she gasped and said, "We need to get outside right now." We went outside and she snapped her fingers above, in front of, and around her body and mine to clear away the negative energy she had felt and she also rushed to the nearby creek to splash a little water over her and me to clear away any negative energy we might have been exposed to. At this point, we decided to walk on up the road for a little while just to get away from the cabin and talk about what she had "felt."

Rahne said that she had felt an "energy" in that particular bedroom that had entered through some sort of portal/vortex that was decidedly negative and seemed as though it had come in through the upstairs window facing the neighbor's cabin next door. The portal/vortex may actually have been closer to our neighbor's cabin. She shared with me that she believed the reason I might have developed schizophrenia in the first place was because I had spent so much time at the cabin in that bedroom during all of the years I had visited while working on my dissertation back in the early to mid-1990s and that I might have been affected by energies traveling in and out of that particular vortex/portal. I remembered that I had always kept the windows open in that bedroom in the cabin. Rahne also shared with me that she thought my aura and energy bodies had been weakened at that time, thus allowing a negative energy or "entity" to "attach." This all sounded very strange and hard to believe, but resonated as truth at the same time because I distinctly remembered a night at the cabin in approximately 1994 or 1995 when, while sleeping, I had what I thought was a very scary nightmare where I saw and felt a dark black force, basically, plunge down and enwrap my head and upper body. I remember waking up from the nightmare and trying to "shake off" the scariness of it. Rahne further explained that she believed negative and dark entities and energies "hang around" places and that people whose auras and energy bodies have become weakened due to alcohol, drugs, stress, etc. might be more easily affected. She recommended staying away from bars, in particular, where many people become drunk which opens up their auras to negative entity attachment.

This same healer friend, Rahne, suggested that I contact the "Raven Clan" to conduct a Raven Wisdom Clearing on me, my home, the cabin, my office work space, my relationships, and my car. I had never heard of the Raven Clan but soon learned that the Ravens are a group of elders/healers who reside in the northwestern part of the United States bordering Canada. At least this particular group did. They have trained and studied for many years and can heal, clear, cleanse, and remove unhealthy entanglements, blocks, entities, etc. remotely. After contacting a correspondent for the Raven clan via email in late April, 2005, I was approved and assigned three clearers who worked on me remotely for 21 days from June 1 to June 21, 2005, each day from 4:00pm until 4:45pm. We needed to wait until June because I was still teaching at the university in May and needed to be available to the Raven Clan clearers/healers in a resting, meditating, or relaxing state as they worked on me from afar. So, each day, from 4:00pm – 4:45pm, I went into my meditation room and either rested, meditated, or listened to a deep relaxation recording. Within minutes, I sensed their presence through hearing creaking at the very tops of the walls in the meditation room. I truly felt they were there and working on me. The idea of being healed remotely or healing others remotely might sound very foreign and downright unbelievable to most readers. I would invite you to do further research on this topic to learn more about this phenomenon.

At the end of the 21 days, I was emailed a fairly lengthy and detailed report of how the clearing went. While keeping the names of the healers/clearers/clan members confidential, I wish now to include specific excerpts from the report that I found incredibly enlightening and fascinating and hope the reader will find informative, too.

The correspondent who communicated to me on behalf of the Raven Clan wrote: "As this was a Level III Clearing, with your input your Raven clearers outlined their work with you to be:

- To clean and sweep all four quadrants (physical, emotional, intellectual-professional, and spiritual), your time-space webbing (past to present to future), and your personal, auric, and etheric fields
- To clear your relational lines with Family of Origin and Family of Choice members, close professional and personal relationships as much as your Higher Self, their Higher Self and Spirit would allow without creating karmic imbalance
- To cleanse and clear your home, cabin, university office space, and vehicle
- To remove any entanglements and blocks found in the under-developed or undeveloped areas of the All-Nourishing Void that could be blocking the progress of publishing your work, your expanding career possibilities in terms of mentoring as well as teaching, your continued creative endeavors, and your creating and sustaining a loving, healthy, reciprocating, long-term male relationship

Your clearers visited, cleared, and cleansed each of these areas before moving into a rather unexpected aspect of their work. When they began their work on your Emotional Quadrant, they discovered that due to trauma approximately a decade ago, soul fragmentation took place in the EQ (Emotional Quadrant) requiring them to find those separated fragmented parts (similar to the soul retrieval process but a bit more complicated since we are speaking of fragments here, not the soul itself) to thus bring the emotional self back into wholeness and balance. The cooperation of your High Self was essential in this last step of soul fragmentation retrieval and, as always, you were most willing to grant permission and access from that realm.

With that overview given, we'll start with the findings from your **Physical Quadrant.** We are pleased to say that this area has been well cared for, plain and simple. The level of toxicity was extremely low due to balanced vigilance over the years with your nutrition, exercise, rest, and release of stressors experienced in everyday life. You are to be commended for this honoring of your physical body. They also worked on each chakra center individually, opening them a bit more fully so that they could function individually and together on a higher vibrational level with greater functionality and balance.

Much to your clearers' surprise, when they entered your **Emotional Quadrant,** they found that in the deeper realms it was very much like a vacuum. That is when they discovered the wounding from trauma that we suspect occurred with your encounter with a multi-dimensional entity at the cabin. Although it was centered around a multi-dimensional, extra-sensory experience, its long term effects on you took place in the EQ (Emotional Quadrant). The Cabin Experience, as your clearers refer to this pivotal point in your growth and development in this incarnation, was as though your EQ was hit by shrapnel and a fragment of your soul was sheared off and spun out into the Void. What your Raven clearers did initially was to change both the frequency and the electro-magnetic charge in this quadrant so that you could once again begin to feel, magnetize, and bring forward into your field that which would energize and complete the healing of what the lead clearer called 'the quiet waiting heart.' What they perceived is that emotionally, on the deeper realms of being, you have felt as though you have been in this quiet waiting mode since the initial healing from the schizophrenia and auditory hallucinations took place after the trauma of the fragmentation. The feeling of stasis and not moving forward or returning back to the past emotionally have been symptoms of the soul fragmentation in the EQ. With this frequency and charge firmly in place, your clearers could then proceed with the process of properly magnetizing the fragment back to the soul and doing the repair and mending necessary for you to have full EQ functioning. This process of healing (repairing/mending) is slow by nature and you should be experiencing the full effects of it over the next three to four months through greater heart connections with self, others, and Spirit, feeling more fully alive, not reviewing the past, not feeling stasis, and beginning to sense other emotional energies that would normally be part of this healthier clustering.

In the **Intellectual-Professional Quadrant,** the Raven Clan clearers found the effects from the vacuum/vacant energy in the Emotional Quadrant having an impact on this quadrant, which would be expected. Such an influence would create a void in your Intellectual-Professional Quadrant in that seeking to manifest service would lead to less than satisfactory results in your perspective time and again. Each effort would be lacking some form of magnetizing force needed to bring into being a more highly integrated system of service in the physical world that accurately reflects the fullness of your wisdom, creativity, and love. We believe that this is the obstacle or force that has stopped publication of your book, which is greatly needed in this world at this time. With the proper energies in place in the EQ, your clearers could then align the I-PQ (Intellectual-Professional Quadrant) with the EQ, remove existing blocks, restructure lines, and move energy into and flowing through this quadrant with grace. As our lead clearer stated, it is a beautiful sight to behold and now the forms of service that Spirit asks you to manifest can come into more satisfying clarity and focus in your intellect and your heart as well as your spirit and thus outwardly into the world, particularly in the form of publication of this great book of yours." (To the reader, the book the Raven Clan correspondent is referring to is the one you are reading at this moment.)

"In the **Spiritual Quadrant,** your clearers felt strongly that you maintain a loving relationship of trust, surrender, and obedience with your Higher Self and Higher Power. They felt humbled to perceive this in action and felt little work needed to be done there to assist you on your earthly journey. It is in right order. Job well done! As always, you could spend a bit more time each day in direct and focused communication with Spirit and maintain more varied modes of Spiritual Discipline.

Your **time-space webbing** indicated that very few repairs and adjustments were needed. The most intense work done here was in putting the parameters into place that will keep you more firmly grounded in the present moment rather than living from a place further down your time-space webbing that we usually call the future. Your time-space webbing indicated that you are highly sensitive to others' fields and absorb a tremendous amount of energies both positive and negative personally and professionally. You also have a somewhat distressing habit of dipping into the Collective, particularly in the dream state. Your clearers placed filters along your webbing and then erected boundaries that would deter only your involuntary trips into the Collective through dream state. Next, your Raven clearers found in your webbing that in being of service to others, you continue to move into a selflessness that has imbalance in that you deplete your own resources within. Your clearers gently remind you to give yourself daily time to renew in giving to others. The point of balance they have set for you is where you give in service while remembering to nurture self.

The **All-Nourishing Void** is the Raven Wisdom teaching term for that area of our being where our potential for growth toward wholeness as well as our shadow aspects reside. It is the area in any clearing that requires the greatest work which is twofold: release the limiters that block our potentiality while clearing and cleansing the shadow aspects (less than affectionately called 'the ugghies'!) that create and recreate debilitating old patterns of behavior. The limiters that were released for you centered on: 1) your fears that your service work will not be in alignment or heard adequately in the world, and 2) your fears that the fullness of your service dreams can indeed become a reality. Therefore, your shadow aspects centered on fears related to manifestation and service, speaking to a powerful underlying sense of non-alignment with this incarnation and the planetary energy, collectively and individually. Again, let me reiterate that the Cabin Experience with the multi-dimensional entity triggered what is generally considered mental illness (i.e. schizophrenia and auditory hallucinations) but this experience also opened the doors to the shadow aspect of self, the ugghies, and the fears. As you have healed yourself, you have been able to feel the pain, injustice, and betrayals of this incarnation and this planet, but have not been fully able to quiet the fears and anxiety that exist within the Deep Self. With the fragments retrieved and knitted back nicely in the EQ, the release and removal of the fears and anxiety then could be addressed by your Raven clearers. This is when you went through the most intense part of the healing crisis. With the permission of the Deep Self, the everyday self, and the High Self plus Spirit's permission, the clearers were allowed to retrieve those fragments, and return and restore them to their proper place within your EQ. With your courage to push through with them, they next were able to release the subtle yet deep hold the fear and anxiety had on aspects of your mind, heart, and spirit. You do have the determination and heart of a spiritual warrior.

The Cabin Experience has had one other major impact on your life: your inability to remain balanced in relationships with men. You either give your trust blindly and then regret it after betrayal, or you fail to give trust in relationships even when it has been earned. Reaching a midpoint of balance between these two behaviors will be far easier to accomplish now – establishing earned trust with men based on your cleared trust in self and Spirit.

We have developed a lovely little mantra to use to continue this renewal of balanced trust in self, others, and Spirit: I surrender, I trust, I am willing, I give, I ask, I receive, I am enough.

In other aspects of your clearing, it became evident to the clearers that you have the heart and soul of the Mentor. In Raven Wisdom teachings, there are eight spiritually-based roles: The Earthsteward, The Artist, The Healer, The Dreamwalker, The Activist, The Mentor, The Sage, and the Seer. You wear the purple color of the Mentor well (each of the roles is color coordinated). The pathway associated with the role is the Path of Inspiration, which means that the criteria for making wise spiritually based choices in your life are: 1) that the choice needs to inspire yourself and 2) be an inspiration to others through your own modeling of a principle, thought, or belief. Whenever the clearers would remove a block or clear an energy line, the darkness of that energy would be replaced again and again with various shadings of purple, violet, fuschia, and what they referred to as 'an awesome amethyst brilliance.'

Although you are familiar with and gifted in other roles, the Mentor continues to be your strength, your service, and your foundation. Secondarily, your spiritual challenge is to develop your Artist role in walking the Pathway of Creative Expression on a deeper and more substantive level. With the clearing process completed, this pathway should be easier to access and work than previously. You had some minor blocks associated with trusting your written communication and those have been cleared as well. The fear limiters mentioned earlier were the major obstacles found on your webbing in terms of publishing your writings.

The clearers were delighted with the results of the soul fragmentation work itself. You hold a strong imprint out there in the Void and finding the aspects set free from earthly bonds went smoothly enough. Restoring them was work very much like putting together the final pieces of a jigsaw puzzle. The lovely part of all this is that your journey toward wholeness will grow much gentler in the process.

Next in the clearing process, the clearers focused on full sweeps of your living space, your vehicle, your work environments, and relational lines to all significant people in your life at present. This work went well enough by your Raven clearers although it required moving more deeply into your past on your time-space webbing and dealt with more karmically oriented lines from earlier in this incarnation and extending through to other incarnations as well.

Within Raven Wisdom teachings, there are 24 Karmic Continuums that center on relationships, which we seek to come to a point of balance on at any time in our incarnation. We generally only work one or two primary continuums and that many secondary continuums as well. Your primary Karmic Continuums for Relationships, from what your clearers could determine, are:

Dependence _____ Interdependence _____ Independence
Self-Love _____ Worthiness _____ Love of Spirit

To grow toward wholeness, we need to experience almost every point on these continuums, which it is believed that we do over many lifetimes until we have experienced all points on all continuums with grace and ease. It is another way of saying that in this way we become Bodhisattvas, evolved enough to move beyond incarnation but choosing to reincarnate to assist and serve humankind in collective evolvement.

Right now, your challenge is to move toward greater **Interdependence** on the first continuum and toward greater **Worthiness** on the second continuum. As we move, we do not leave behind the lessons learned and disciplines gained from other points on the continuums. We incorporate those experiences in with what we are learning as you move, in your case, toward understanding, embracing and living Interdependence with others with an increased sense of Worthiness that will manifest in abundance, joy, and acceptance of the gifts of grace.

Anything energetically that stood in the way of movement toward these points on your two continuums was removed with permission sought and granted from your Higher Self and from Spirit.

One last point here, Karma is not viewed in Raven Wisdom teachings as connections between individuals over lifetimes but imbalances we experience within ourselves during incarnations that individuals contract to assist us with through positive and negative life experiences. Your karmic lines of contracts with individuals who no longer are assisting you with learning true Worthiness and Interdependence were disconnected with great care by your clearers who also placed a new set of filters so that you can magnetize a higher frequency of healthfulness and growth within your students, your evolving Family of Choice and in terms of a new paradigm for male relationships.

Relational lines to those whom you hold most dearly in this life were cleared of the energies that create disharmony, misunderstanding, and dependency. As always, the lines between you and your very chaotic Family of Origin were a complex webbing that were untangled with the utmost delicacy. The lines between you and most family members required little to no work once untangled. Most often these family members were seeking something from you that you are not in this life to give them. Their perception of you may never align with your reality but your understanding of this assists you in moving through and beyond it. In most instances, your clearers felt strongly that repeated contact with them would be detrimental to your continued spiritual evolution, emotional growth, and overall balance.

Your living space was essentially in good shape but needed cleansing and clearing in one area specifically, which was in the east central upward quadrant, that held a negative residue that was draining productivity, enhancing self-doubt, and, most importantly, disturbing the harmony and the sense of sanctuary your home offers you. The remainder of the living space held charged yet positive energy overall. If you can bring more light physically into this upper east central space where the negative residue was removed, this would be a most positive and welcome change that will impact your adjacent home office as well.

In addition to this one negative residue in your living space located adjacent to your home office, your clearers also discovered the presence of a more ancient energy in the form of a confluence of energy grids that exists near your university work office. In Raven teachings, Travelers are entities who rather impersonally come and go through dimensions and space, using the confluence of gridding as their rest stop between and among realms and planes. Without going into too much unnecessary detail, your Raven clearers and two other Raven members, shifted the gridding enough so that your present university office space will now be bypassed by multi-dimensional Travelers for a much more stable grid confluence.

They felt it was a much easier solution than trying to erect and maintain 'No Trespassing' signs and boundaries metaphysically speaking for the Travelers. This grid-shift took place six days ago and has been holding steady and firm ever since. One of the clearers commented on how often he found such gridding arrangements in our public buildings and other busy impersonal areas where we work, shop, and gather collectively. It's fascinating to think that we as humans construct our physical public buildings oftentimes over these multi-dimensional public grids!

Your vehicle needs to be checked on the physical level for a minor problem that could manifest in the days ahead. Please have the large belt that circles your engine checked for cracks. Your clearers noted that this belt's energy had reached the end of its useful life. Your tires appear to be fine but you have one water hose that needs to be looked at. They also noticed that you are an easily distracted driver and suggest that you keep your attention more present-moment oriented when driving for safety's sake. I guess you gave them a bit of a fright on more than one occasion when you were elsewhere while driving.

As for other aspects of your work environment, the Raven clearers untangled lines and cleared relatively minor blocks so that you could work at your most creative and productive. Both work spaces, at home and at the university, were cleaned and cleared thoroughly of any toxicity and residue on any realm, either covert or latent. They found both offices abounding in flow and joyous expression that sometimes were a bit too undirected or scattered. Your clearers thoroughly enjoyed working with you to assist in bringing greater focus, clarity, and direction to your creative mentoring endeavors. They loved your energy and enthusiasm for so many different types of expression! One clearer stated that he felt you have clearly heard the call to express yourself creatively through your writing and that your greatest challenge is to move forward with trust in your message to the world."

After receiving the report from the Raven Clan clearers, I was given the opportunity to ask questions about any part of the report. I asked the clearers if it was now safe to go back to the cabin since I had always enjoyed visiting there. Also, at this time, a huge forest fire was blazing through the national forest on which our family cabin is built. Due to the fire, 11 of the 44 cabins had burned to the ground. Our cabin was saved, but the cabin that was ten feet beside us had burned down. As mentioned earlier, my Raven Clan healing/clearing occurred from June

1 through June 21 between 4:00pm and 4:45pm each day. The final day of clearing was June 21, 2005, at 4:45pm. In researching the cause of the fire on the national forest where the cabins are located, I found out online that the fire was believed to have started due to a lightning strike from a thunderstorm. The date and time the online website identified for the beginning of the fire was June 21, 2005, at 4:45pm. I could hardly believe my eyes when I read this. I shared the start date and time of the fire with the correspondent for the clearers.

In answer to my question regarding safely visiting the cabin, the correspondent for the Raven Clan clearers explained:

"About the cabin: It is safe for you now to go back up to the cabin. The multi-dimensional entity can no longer affect you since it was finally removed from that area on June 21st. Therefore, it would be safe for the rest of the family to go up there as well. I wonder without ever knowing the answer if the fire is somehow related to the removal of that particular entity along with several others in that area that the Ravens found while doing their work with you. As you know, entities create electro-magnetic disturbances, some of which can result in fire. If this indeed did happen, then we have to look at the fire as a cleansing before renewal as we often find with Gaia (Greek mythology's Divine Mother)."

SEARCH FOR MY FAMILY OF CHOICE

After learning so much from the Raven Clan clearers and feeling so much better about life, I wanted to learn even more about how I could increase my circle of friends and family that would or could become, as the Ravens called it, my "Family of Choice." This "family" had already begun to manifest back in 2004 when I felt guided to reconnect with a childhood friend, Mary Ann. We visited together when I attended an educational conference in Florida, connected again when she and a friend traveled west in 2004, and she came to visit me in Arizona for about a week in 2005. We have so many common beliefs and interests and she is a wonderful support in my life. The downside was that she lived and continues to live in Florida and we do not get to see each other as often as we would like. But, we talk on the phone at least twice a month and are regularly in contact via email.

It was also during this time that I decided to read and learn more about areas in life in which I would like to grow. I thought that, by learning more, I might make better choices in connecting with others of "like mind" who might become future family members of choice. I started by reading a book that I seemed to be "led to" in a bookstore called *God, Creation, and Tools for Life* by Sylvia Browne. By reading this book, my mind was opened up to a whole new way of thinking about God and spirituality. Sylvia not only writes in depth about the concepts of a father and mother God and numerous levels of the Soul, but she also provides what she calls "Tools for Life" for the reader to use to transform negative energy, utilize lights and colors, and protect against psychic attack including the use of positive affirmations. I list many of Sylvia Browne's books in the references and recommended reading section included at the end of this book.

MEDITATION GROUP

In the fall of 2005, I began searching for and trying out various prayer and meditation groups in town in order to connect with more like minded people. I attended a prayer group led by Dr. Cay Randall-May, the medical intuitive that originally worked on me in the early stages of my schizophrenia and referred me directly to my family doctor. I wrote about her earlier in this book and will write more about her later. She is an amazing, highly educated, and spiritually minded lady!

Next, I learned about a group that was purportedly studying the hidden meaning of life. While I did learn a great deal while attending this group once a week for approximately two months, it didn't feel like "home" to me, so I searched further. In December, 2005, I attended a workshop on "Starpeople" offered at a local new age bookstore. At the end of the workshop, the presenter, Miguel Montoya, invited us to begin attending his newly-forming meditation group which was to meet weekly there at the bookstore. I began attending right away and a small group of us became good friends. We spent quite a bit of time together outside of the meditation group meetings. We went on road trips to fun and spiritual places, went to movies, and out to dinners. The meditation group and our friendships continued over the next few years. I had the entire group over to my house for potluck dinners and parties several times. I began feeling so much better about life.

During the first half of the year 2006, I found myself more involved socially which contributed to improved self-esteem, greater friendships, and positive spiritual growth. My career was going well and I even began dating again. A very special friend I had made when I was an educational consultant who, in 2006, was teaching for me part time in my university undergraduate education program, called one day to ask if I would like to come to a dinner party she and her husband were having because she had met a single man at another couple's cookout who she would like for me to meet. She really thought we would hit it off. I was just getting ready to go on a short vacation to visit family in Texas, but told her I would love to attend her dinner party when I returned. It was at this dinner party in mid-2006 that I met Scott Stackhouse, the true love of my life.

FINDING TRUE LOVE

At the dinner party given by my friend, Dona, and her husband, Mark, were two other married couples and my future husband and me. Scott and I did hit it off right away as Dona had predicted and we talked nonstop throughout the evening. At the end of the party, Scott asked for my telephone number and he walked me to my car. He called the next day and asked if he could go with me to the meditation group I had been attending (I had told him about this group during the dinner party) and then take me out to his favorite Mexican food restaurant. I said yes! We had a wonderful time and I was so happy to know that he was interested in spirituality and meditation. We had many other things in common. He was 53 and I was 50 so we were fairly close in age. We both liked the same music although he introduced me to various classic rock groups and I introduced him to more new age and Native American music. We both liked to travel and go on "road trips." From 2006 until 2008, we went to many different restaurants, attended meditation group, met each other's parents, went to musical concerts, traveled, met each other's family members and friends, spent a great deal of time with each other, and fell in love.

Professionally in our careers, we both worked very hard, but I think Scott had to spend more time working than I did. He had a fulltime job in outdoor commercial and residential landscape design, installation, and maintenance and also a part time job doing interior commercial and residential plant design, installation, and maintenance. I continued working fulltime as a university professor in education and enjoying it immensely. If there was any fault I could find in him or the relationship, it was that he worked too hard and was not available as often as I would have liked, although, when I look back at all of the places we went and time we spent together, I think we have done so much more together than many other people and couples we know. I tried to keep up with my own interests including exercising, seeing girlfriends, spending time with my mom, visiting the cabin, and attending meditation groups. The group Scott and I were both involved in had disbanded because the group leader, Miguel, moved to another city. The lightbody healer friend I mentioned earlier had emailed me information about another local meditation group she had heard wonderful things about. I decided to give the other group a try and have been attending whenever I can since 2006 all the way to the present 2012.

COSMIC TRAVELS HEALING AND MEDITATION GROUP

It has been a blessed experience to attend this special mediation group where each member is thought of as a gifted healer, lightworker, artist, psychic, channeler, and/or medium. The group meets every Thursday evening. The first meeting of each month has been and continues to be dedicated to "healing circle" where everyone gets a chance to receive, give, and use their healing talents. Since I had learned Usui and Mahatma Reiki in the past, I contribute this healing art whenever I attend healing circle. (Additionally, I have very recently been trained as a Transdimensional Reiki Master). The other weeks of the month are dedicated to guided meditation, group healing, and channeling facilitated primarily by Melissa Galka, the female leader of the group. She and her husband, John Galka, both sometimes channel the "Language of Light" (the reader might wish to research this topic). I have also had the honor and benefit of personal healing sessions directed and channeled by Melissa. She has opened up my mind to many different healing modalities and has assisted me in clearing out past life trauma, issues, and cellular memories that needed to be released. She is also a medium and has connected to special people in my life that have passed over including my Aunt Juanita and my brother, Steve, who I have mentioned so often in this book. I will talk a little more about Melissa and the meditation group in the next chapter as they are very important in helping me to maintain balance in all parts of my life.

The reason it is so important to have been guided to this particular meditation group is because I always feel so accepted there. I believe there are many members in the group who have more faith in my spiritual, healing, and psychic abilities than I do. Melissa mentioned to me early on and again recently that she thought I should develop my own abilities as a psychic medium. As you might remember from earlier in this book, I was able to connect with my brother, Steve, on the other side after he had just taken his own life but before I even heard here on the earth plane that he had passed. When the father of my now husband, Scott, passed in 2007, I was able to connect with him as well and share his messages with his wife (my husband's mother) and son, Scott. The seed was planted for me to actually do something with this gift.

However, at this point, between 2006 and 2008, I was going strong in my academic career teaching pre-service teachers how to become elementary school teachers. Next, I will briefly describe two very different events that occurred near the end of 2008 that were highly emotional and have dramatically changed my life.

A DECEMBER TO REMEMBER

The year 2008 had been such a wonderful year for Scott and me full of fun people and activities including: 1) our travel to Florida to see my childhood friend, Mary Ann (the one I mentioned earlier in this chapter of having reconnected with) and her fiancé, Jeff, 2) our standing up for her and Jeff during their April wedding in Sedona, Arizona, 3) going on many road trips together, and 4) even spending time together at our family cabin. We continued to attend many musical events and concerts and spend time with each other's families. Earlier in 2008, my favorite Aunt Juanita who was 85 years old began to suffer from a failing heart. She was placed in the hospital for a time, but was soon able to go home. This favorite aunt of mine was the one I mentioned earlier in the book who was responsible for inspiring my move to Arizona. At this point, I had lived in Arizona for 30 years and had spent the majority of my holidays as well as other times throughout the year seeing her or spending time with her. Over the past two years, since meeting Scott, we had spent time together especially at Thanksgiving and Christmas. She loved Scott and felt we were a fantastic match. He totally loved her, too.

The last time we spent with Aunt Juanita was to meet my Mom and Aunt for lunch early in December, 2008. Scott brought Aunt Juanita a poinsettia, but we could all tell she was not doing well. Within the next few days, she was back in the hospital for the last time. She hung on for two days, but passed on December 11, 2008. I kept her last Christmas card that she sent to us which she must have written and sent the day before she went into the hospital. She wrote to me, "I do appreciate you so much, all the nice things you do for me," and to Scott, "Thank you so very much – the poinsettia is beautiful! You are very kind and thoughtful to me. Love to you." The funeral was very hard and sad for us both. Scott served as a pall bearer and was so honored to do so. We both miss her very much and talk about her often. She was quite a character and I connect with her sometimes on the other side. I often ask her for advice and I hear her answers. I also feel she is visiting when butterflies are around.

My aunt, unfortunately, had passed before I became engaged to the love of my life. Scott proposed on Christmas Eve of 2008 and presented me with the most amazing and beautiful diamond engagement ring I've ever seen! Of course, I said yes!! We celebrated the next day, Christmas Day, with my mom and had a wonderful Christmas dinner at a local resort.

At this point in my life, I had almost completely forgotten that I ever had depression and schizophrenia. They were both so very far behind me now. This was a wonderful place for me to be. However, it is important to note, at this point, the many additional gifts that I had been blessed with that brought me to this place.

MORE GIFTS

1. Lightbody activations
2. More books
3. Raven Clan Wisdom Clearing
4. Expanding my family of choice
5. Cosmic Travels Healing and Meditation Group
6. Finding my true love, Scott, and getting engaged

Before going on to the final chapter of this book, I would like to offer the reader time to reflect on aspects of his or her own life related to the information discussed within this chapter.

READER'S WORKBOOK: HEALING EXPERIENCES
AND HEALTHY RELATIONSHIPS

1. What healing experiences (both traditional and non-traditional) have you been blessed with in your life?

_____

_____

_____

_____

_____

_____

_____

_____

_____

_____

_____

_____

_____

2. Name two or three books related to healing that you have read recently that have had a positive or enlightening effect on you.

_____

_____

_____

_____

_____

_____

_____

_____

_____

_____

_____

_____

_____

_____

_____

_____

_____

3. What, if any, parts of the Raven Clan clearing report were interesting to you or could you resonate with?

_____

_____

_____

_____

_____

_____

_____

_____

_____

_____

_____

_____

_____

_____

_____

4. Describe positive relationships you hold with two or three
    family of origin (biological family) members. Explain why these
    relationships are healthy and reciprocal.

_____

_____

_____

_____

_____

_____

_____

_____

_____

_____

_____

_____

_____

5. Describe negative relationships you hold with two or three family of origin members. Describe any aspects of the relationships that are unhealthy.

_____

_____

_____

_____

_____

_____

_____

_____

_____

_____

_____

_____

_____

_____

_____

6. Describe any healthy relationships you have chosen with those people who are in your family of choice as explained in this chapter. Why did you choose these people as family of choice members? Have these relationships made your life healthier and happier? Explain.

_____

_____

_____

_____

_____

_____

_____

_____

_____

_____

_____

_____

_____

_____

7. What community or spiritual groups do you belong to that nurture your authentic self and leave you feeling accepted and happy?

_____

_____

_____

_____

_____

_____

_____

_____

_____

_____

_____

_____

_____

_____

_____

8. Have you been blessed with finding the love of your life? If so, explain how this person blesses your life. If not, make a list of ten characteristics you are looking for in the true love of your life.

_____

_____

_____

_____

_____

_____

_____

_____

_____

_____

_____

_____

_____

_____

_____

_____

_____

CHAPTER NINE

Maintaining the Balance and Staying Positive

A t this point, I had begun to feel as though my life had true balance between work, play, scholarship, exercise, spirituality, romance, relationships, finance, and other aspects of my life. My self-esteem was high and I seemed to be smiling all of the time. My life was flowing in a positive direction and I wanted to maintain this strong and positive balance I had achieved. The thought of ever having had depression or schizophrenia was non-existent. Earlier in chapter five, I mentioned that my psychiatrist once explained to me that the best indicator of having been cured of schizophrenia is not remembering that I ever had it. I was finally there!

As 2009 began, my fiancé, Scott, and I began making plans for our new life together. We started with putting my house up for sale so that I would be able to move into the house he had (and we currently have). We placed my house on the market in April, the same month I earned a solid and well compensated promotion at the university, and, by June, the house was sold with a small profit earned. Our wedding date was set and plans were beginning for our upcoming wedding.

WEDDING BELLS

By April, 2009, we had scheduled our wedding at a beautiful golf course venue in Scottsdale, Arizona. The wedding date was early November, 2009. We each chose our best friends to stand up for us (Mary and Warren). I couldn't believe that, at age 53, I was picking out my first wedding dress with my best friend, Mary, at my side. It was so much fun to attend the local bridal show and get so excited about all of the wedding plans! At the bridal show, I won a free engagement sitting and a free limousine ride (which Scott and I used to go to the airport as we left for our honeymoon). My fiancé and I soon picked out all of the colors, flowers, photographer, cake, everything!

The person we decided to have officiate at the wedding was Reverend Cay Randall-May. She was the medical intuitive I had consulted originally at the very beginnings of my symptoms of schizophrenia. I wrote about her earlier in chapter two. I had also regularly attended her Sunday Prayer Circles for a while and my fiancé had met her, too. She was happy to "marry" us and met with us a few times before the wedding to provide counseling and advice. I had read her book *The Intuitive Career: How to Succeed as a Consultant, Reader, or Healer* and she gave us her most recent publication *Healing and the Creative Response: Four Key Steps Shared by Healers and Artists* as a wedding gift. I have listed these two books in the references and recommended reading section at the end of this book.

We invited approximately 70 family members and friends to our wedding. My fiancé, Scott, had the inspired idea of setting up a special table with photos in the reception hall to commemorate those who had passed on and were so special to us. They included my brother, Steve Duke, my aunt, Juanita Ingalls, Scott's father, Jacques Stackhouse, Scott's grandfather, Truman Davis, Scott's grandmother, Fern Davis, my grandmother, Luella Abbott, my grandfather, Nolan Abbott, and my grandmother, Blanche Duke. Those still living included my mom and my dad who were both able to attend. At the age of 76, my dad, Frank Duke, even walked me down the aisle. I was so thrilled he was able to be there. My dad and my Uncle Eddie (my dad's younger brother) drove all the way from Florida to attend. Scott's mother, Cherie Stackhouse from Denver, Colorado, and most of our siblings and family members were able to share in our happy wedding day. Many of our close friends and co-workers came to see us get married including the couple who introduced us. I was especially thankful that my friend, Jackie, was there.

She is such a wise, insightful, supportive, and positive person in my life. She is truly a guardian angel to me, her family, and many others. Jackie's granddaughter, Alexa, then five years old, was our beautiful little flower girl.

The outdoor wedding was perfect, the music was amazing, the food was delicious, and I believe everyone had a great time! We left the next morning for a week long honeymoon in Cancun and Playa del Carmen, Mexico. On our honeymoon, we stayed in a beautiful condominium with a rooftop Jacuzzi and view of the ocean. We went to the beach, visited Chichen Itza, saw many other sites, and had a marvelous time. We were very much in love and life was good! While we were on our honeymoon, whenever I had time alone to think, I would replay and relive the entire wedding in my mind, and, while flying home from our honeymoon, I would, again, replay and relive the entire wedding and honeymoon over and over. I was so happy to have had these blessings in my life. Even today, if I get a little down, one of my favorite ways to cheer myself up is to look at all of our wedding and honeymoon photographs.

MARRIAGE, TRAVEL, FUN!

Because my husband and I truly do have so much in common, we have enjoyed many fun times together both before marriage and after. We love music and concerts. Some of the musical artists and groups we've been fortunate to see have included The Doobie Brothers, Heart, Chris Botti, Deva Premal and Miten, Al Stewart, Carlos Nakai, Crosby, Stills, and Nash, America, Loggins and Messina, David Gray, Dave Mason, Tom Petty, Johnny Rivers, Nils Lofgren, Sarah MacLachlin, War, and Wilco. We like going out for dinners and movies. We have a family cabin that I have mentioned several times in this book that we like to go to every so often just to relax, light a fire in the fireplace, hike outside in the national forest, and eat good food. We also enjoy day trips and have visited some fun and beautiful places here in Arizona. More distant travel we have experienced together has included Colorado, California, and Florida.

Since neither one of us has children, we have been fairly free to do many things we love to do. My husband has a true and artistic love for landscaping, so, not only does our yard look beautiful and magical, but we like to visit local gardens and arboretums whenever we can. I love going for walks and attending meditation and healing groups and my husband will accompany me once in a while. We both have recently discovered that we have an interest in UFOs, extra-terrestrials, and ancient alien sites here on planet Earth and we regularly attend lectures and presentations at a local mutual unidentified flying objects network. We don't necessarily believe in all that we have heard, but it is fun and interesting!

While we have been very blessed in trying to focus on our commonalities and the positive parts of marriage and learning to blend and merge together as a couple, I must admit that, in several ways, it has been quite an adjustment for both of us during these first few years of marriage.

ADJUSTING TO MARRIAGE – THE HARD PARTS

Soon after our honeymoon, my husband, Scott, and I began having disagreements and arguments mostly about my perception that he was too busy to spend quality time together and/or to plan fun things for us to do together. We both work fulltime jobs. The hours I work for my university job are much more flexible than the hours he works in landscape supervision and maintenance. I teach in the evenings and can work from my home computer and telephone a few days a week and can also work from home to grade papers and call into meetings. My husband does not have those luxuries and, most days, needs to awaken by 4:00am in order to get to work early to get all of his crews going to their job sites. Scott is on the go and on the phone pretty much non-stop throughout the day and spends much of his time visiting high end residential sites to be sure the quality of the work is excellent. He usually doesn't arrive home until 5:30pm and needs to get to bed by 8:00pm during the week to get adequate sleep. Since I frequently teach until 10:00pm at night and get home by 10:30pm, my sleeping hours are usually from 11:00pm until 7:00am during the week. So, as you might imagine, our work hours have proven to be a bit of an obstacle (at least for me). My husband also works a second job part-time doing interior plant work for offices, primarily. He has to fit this in during the week and on weekends. I, also, once or twice a year, am called to participate in visits to underperforming or failing schools in our state for two to three days each, basically, to perform an audit of the school along with other team members and create a report of findings and recommendations for improvement for the school we are visiting.

During our first year of marriage, we did have numerous disagreements and arguments over the issue of not having enough time together and we went so far as to attend counseling sessions with two different therapists. One therapist gave each of us excellent advice including, for me, to try not to control everything so much and to try to understand and accept my husband's schedule and personality more, and, for my husband, to try to take the work "hat" off when he gets home and to be sure to plan activities that I might like to do. This first therapist also taught us quite a bit about the "Five Love Languages" and how each of us might prefer to be shown love differently. The second therapist recommended the actual book entitled *The Five Love Languages* by Chapman. She also recommended a second book entitled *How to Improve Your Marriage without Talking About It* by Love and Stosny. We each have read both books, they have helped quite a bit, and I have listed them in the references and recommended reading list at the end of the book.

Another strategy we tried for the first two years of our marriage was to have what we called "Daytimer Meetings" where we would bring our daytimers to a meeting at our dining room table on Sundays and talk about and schedule the upcoming week and sometimes special events for the month. Many times, these meetings led to further disagreements and arguments. What we have finally been able to compromise on includes: 1) picking one night during the week to be together where we have a deep relaxation, make dinner at home, and then do something fun like play a game of billiards, watch a television show, or listen to some music, 2) planning some fun events for weekends and holidays and writing them on our calendars, and 3) identifying at least one weekend a month for unplanned or spontaneous time together. Sometimes, I write out a list of what we are doing for the week including the times and I leave this for my husband in our kitchen drawer. This last strategy has helped a great deal in reducing our disagreements and/or arguments. I think I have learned that he needs time to read the list, digest it, work it into his very busy schedule, and let me know if something will not work. I have to say that he tries very, very hard to include everything. I am trying harder to not ask for so much of his time and I have noticed that, the less time I ask of him, the more he seems to want to find time to be together.

We have also learned that we truly want to be each other's best friend and we try to check in with each other every so often to see if we are accomplishing this. We are both very independent people and we're learning how to be, as the Raven Clan clearers would say, interdependent. I think, finally, and most recently, we are learning and practicing the fine and complicated art of "not pushing each other's buttons." We are both learning that it helps to keep in mind the idea that we should try harder to be patient and compassionate with each other. It has also helped me to ask myself, when my buttons might be pushed, "How can I best react to this situation that would be in a mature and grown-up manner?" Sometimes, Scott or I ask for a timeout to calm down, regroup, and come back together with a more collected and positive attitude. This, of course, is easier said than done! I've also asked Scott to please say, "Yes, dear" a little more often This has helped, too! And, as an update, Scott was recently successful in returning back to the company he left one and a half years ago. We can both already tell that he is much, much happier there and he will always get to sleep until at least 5:30am or 6:00am! What a huge gift to each of us and to our marriage!

All in all, I think we are both at a point in our marriage and in our lives where we truly do know that we love each other very much and want to spend the rest of our lives together. We had waited until our 50s to find each other and realize that loving each other is a choice we need to wake up and make each and every day. This leads me to a discussion of the differences between the families we each are born into and the families we end up choosing to be with over the course of our lives.

FAMILY OF ORIGIN VS. FAMILY OF CHOICE

As explained in chapter eight, there is a difference between one's family of origin and family of choice. Each person's family of *origin* includes his or her biological family (parents, grandparents, brothers, sisters, etc.). An individual's family of *choice* would or could include both biological family members and friends who resonate closely with a person's own vibrational frequency. Portions of the Raven Clan Wisdom Clearing Report were included in chapter eight and, as a review, described my own family of origin as chaotic and comprised of family members who were seeking something from me that I am not in this life to give them. The Raven Clan report went on to say that most of my biological family members' perceptions of me may never align with my true reality, but my understanding of this assists me in moving through and beyond it. In most instances, my Raven Clan clearers felt strongly that repeated contact with certain members of my biological family or family of origin would be detrimental to my continued spiritual evolution, emotional growth, and overall balance.

The reason I am reviewing this information here is because, over the past six to seven years since the Raven Clan Wisdom Clearing, I definitely feel as though I have disconnected with or continue to move towards more of a disconnect status with many biological family of origin members. More accurately, I believe many or most of them have decided to disconnect from me. For years, I have tried to maintain contact with several family members, but our lives really are so different that it seems we truly do not have very much in common anymore. This is okay. My meditation group leader, Melissa, describes her family of origin members as previous roommates at college. It was fun when they were together and the times together served a purpose, but now, all have graduated and moved on to other interests and other lives that do not intersect with hers anymore.

I believe this is the same with me. As explained earlier by the Raven Clan clearers, karma is not viewed in Raven Wisdom teachings as connections between individuals over lifetimes, but imbalances we experience within ourselves during incarnations that individuals (both family of origin members and others in life) contract to assist us with through positive and negative life experiences. My karmic lines of contracts with individuals who no longer are assisting me with learning true worthiness and interdependence were disconnected with great care by my clearers. This has proven to be a wonderful blessing to me.

The very good news is that I have been and continue to develop an amazing family of choice that resonates with my vibrational frequency. This does not mean that family of origin members with whom I have either limited or no contact are viewed by me as better or worse. It just means that we have different life paths, purposes, and interests. My life path, purpose, and interests now include attracting and interacting with family of choice members who are positive, respectful, honest, healthful, and with whom I can interdependently grow spiritually, intellectually, and emotionally and with whom I can find balance in not giving too much of myself so that I am depleted, but being open to receiving as well. Some of my very special family of choice members include: my husband, Scott Stackhouse, my best friend of 26 years, Mary Krening, who lives here in Arizona, my childhood friend, Mary Ann Schumacher, who lives in Florida, my friend, Jackie Earnhart, who lives in California, my brother-in-law, John Ensworth, and sister-in-law, Priscilla Clark, who live in Texas, my university colleague of six years, Toni Rantala, and a few others. I am extremely blessed. I have learned so very much from all of these "family of choice" members. I look forward to adding additional "family of choice" members to my life and hope to become members of others' "families of choice" as well.

I believe it is still important to learn from one's "family of origin" and I will always count the many blessings I have had just because I was born into my particular family. I have mentioned many of those blessings in previous chapters of this book. Furthermore, both my husband and I have been and continue to be very interested in finding out more about our own heritages, cultures, and backgrounds and, in August of 2011, experienced an incredible two week dream trip to Scotland and Ireland which I will share about next.

SCOTLAND/IRELAND TRIP

My cultural ancestry includes Irish, Scotch Irish, English, Dutch, German, and Native American. My husband's ancestry includes English, possibly Scottish, and French. Early in our marriage we made a list of places we would like to visit as a couple before we pass on. Those places we listed included Ireland and Scotland, New Zealand and Australia, Peru and the Galapagos Islands, Greece and Italy, Prince Edward Island, and British Columbia. My husband was kind enough to let me pick the destination of our first "big trip." I chose Scotland and Ireland. After much research and deciding that we did not want to practice driving on the left hand side of the road, we opted for a guided coach tour of the two countries. The benefits of this choice included not having to drive, getting to meet and travel with approximately 45 other people, and seeing as many sights as possible. The only downside we found was that we did not get enough time to slow down a little and relax and enjoy the magnificent hotels in which we stayed.

The trip was approximately two weeks in length. We flew into Glasgow, Scotland, and visited and stayed in Glasgow, Nairn, and Edinburgh (all in Scotland). We explored the amazing Kelvingrove Art Museum, Loch Lomond, Urquhart Castle by Loch Ness, a Scottish whisky distillery, and Edinburgh Castle. We attended the Military Tattoo, saw Scottish dancers and musicians, and sampled several Scottish pubs. After ferrying over to Larne, Ireland, we toured Belfast and stayed in Dublin, Killarney, and Shannon (all in Ireland). In Dublin, we visited Trinity College where we viewed the Book of Kells, an illuminated manuscript of gospels created by monks during the 8th century, the Guinness Storehouse (seven stories high!), and attended an Irish dinner theater. We saw the Rock of Cashel, kissed the Blarney stone at Blarney Castle where we also saw some beautiful fern gardens, and shopped and ate lunch at the Blarney Woollen Mills. We visited the Skellig Island Experience, saw a farmer and sheepdog demonstration, and traveled along the picturesque Ring of Kerry. One of our favorite places was Killarney National Park. Again, we visited some pubs warm with music, good cheer, and good food. A highlight of the trip was seeing the spectacular Cliffs of Moher. The trip concluded at Bunratty Castle near Shannon where we enjoyed an authentic medieval feast complete with entertainment. We both agreed that Ireland was our favorite of the two countries and we had a fabulous time overall.

It was so fun visiting places that were new to both of us. We learned so much about the wonderful Scottish and Irish cultures and people. We are also very grateful that we have manifested good jobs, salaries, and health so we can continue to travel more. We plan to have a big trip such as this once every two years. We already have our list of places to go and I think Peru and the Galapagos Islands will be our next destinations since, my husband gets to choose this one, and, by the time we go, we will be a couple of years older (57 and 61), but still young and active enough to adjust to and successfully navigate the high altitudes of Machu Picchu in Peru (we hope!).

I know that I, personally, have found it very effective to write down not only all of the things for which I am grateful but also future goals I wish to manifest or achieve in life which leads me to a discussion of how important gratitude and positive affirmations are in changing all areas and facets of my life and yours for the better.

IMPORTANCE OF GRATITUDE AND POSITIVE AFFIRMATIONS

Back in chapter two of this book, I talked about the importance of taking time to identify all of the wonderful things to be grateful for in our lives. And, in chapter six, I talked about how we can each "do this life" on planet Earth better and you, the reader, had the opportunity to list some ideas of how you would like to improve the various areas of your life such as self-esteem, family relationships, friends, romance, health, body image, work/career, finances, continuing education, spiritual growth, service to the planet, expressing creativity, and more. I also asked the reader to choose only two or three of the areas to focus on and begin to make plans to implement some of your ideas for improvement in your life. Now, at this point in the book, I would like to share with the reader an effective strategy I have read and learned about from Doreen Virtue and Louise Hay. Both of these authors as well as many others have written extensively about the use of positive affirmations to change our lives for the better by changing how we think about what it is we want to manifest or bring into our lives.

Two books, in particular, that I would like to mention, both written by Louise Hay, are *Heal Your Body A-Z: The Mental Causes for Physical Illness and the Way to Overcome Them* and *I Can Do It: How to Use Affirmations to Change Your Life*. Both books teach us how to identify particular thought patterns that may have led us to certain challenges which, while sometimes uncomfortable and debilitating, in actuality, are opportunities for self-healing and growth. An example Louise provides in her *Heal Your Body A-Z* book is that if I am suffering from neck problems, the probable mental cause or thought form I am holding might be "refusing to see other sides of a question, stubbornness, or inflexibility" and the new thought form or positive affirmation I might use to overcome this inflexibility might be to say aloud or to myself: "It is with flexibility and ease that I see all sides of an issue. There are endless ways to do things and see things. I am safe." Louise gives many other examples for ailments listed A-Z with probable causes and new thought patterns. I need to emphasize that Louise Hay does not believe that the probable causes of the physical illnesses or the thinking that may have led to them is at all "bad." She does not believe it is healthy to judge ourselves as wrong, but to view the situation or health challenge we find ourselves in as an opportunity to apply new thinking that will assist in training our minds to manifest physical health. I have also read two other books by Louise Hay: *You Can Heal Your Life* and *Inner Wisdom: Meditations for the Heart and Soul* and they are listed in the references and recommended reading section at the end of this book.

In her book *I Can Do It*, which I have read only recently, Louise explains, "Every thought you think and every word you speak is an affirmation. You are affirming and creating your life experiences with every word and thought." Furthermore, she discusses topics such as health, forgiveness, prosperity, creativity, relationships, job success, stress-free living, and self-esteem and provides numerous positive affirmations to assist in changing these areas of life for the better.

The following are several positive affirmations I have been using from Louise's books to help me maintain my balance, stay positive, and make wonderful changes in my life:

Health: "I enjoy the foods that are best for my body. I love every cell of my body," and "My body is always doing its best to create perfect health."

Forgiveness: "I cannot change another person. I let others be who they are, and I simply love who I am," and "I am forgiving, loving, gentle, and kind, and I know that life loves me."

Prosperity: "I radiate success, and prosper wherever I turn," and "I delight in the financial security that is constant in my life."

Creativity: "There is ample time and opportunity for creative expression in whatever area I choose," and "I create easily and effortlessly when I let my thoughts come from the loving space of my own heart."

Love and Romance (Relationships): "My partner is the love of my life. We adore each other," and "I am safe in all my relationships, and I give and receive lots of love."

Job Success: "My job allows me to express my talents and abilities, and I am grateful for this employment," and "The perfect job is looking for me, and we are being brought together now."

Stress-Free Living: "I let go of all fear and doubt, and life becomes simple and easy for me," and "I slowly breathe in and out, and I find myself relaxing more and more with each breath."

Self-Esteem: "My self-esteem is high because I honor who I am," and "Life supports me in every possible way."

There are many, many other positive affirmations written in Louise's books, but those mentioned above have been effective for me. I have noticed great improvements in my 1) relationship with my husband, 2) zest for life with regard to my current career as a university professor, 3) development of a happier, more positive, and powerful self-esteem, 4) ability to forgive others and myself, and 5) inspiration to creatively express myself in the writing and completion of this book.

Next, I want to share with the reader a process I use to manifest my goals. I will identify two goals I currently have and write positive affirmations to make them a reality in my life.

FUTURE GOALS

I believe we each want to feel good every day, get excited about goals we set, and stay engaged with life in order to fulfill our earthbound purposes. I also believe that it is extremely important to be in gratitude for all we have. Earlier in this book, I mentioned that I identify ten things to be grateful for before I go to sleep at night. This is also a wonderful strategy to use when you first awaken to get started on a positive note in the morning. A gratitude list can also be thought of as a list of gifts to be thankful for. Throughout this book, I have taken time to list all of the many different gifts I have been blessed with throughout my life. Even an illness such as schizophrenia can be thought of as a gift for me because of all the opportunities for growth that have resulted from it. A gratitude or gift list validates and solidifies in my mind what I have gone through, what I have achieved, and what I am thankful for, but, more importantly, keeps me in a positive frame of mind that can support and maintain my health and joy.

Even though I am currently 56 years old, I hope to healthfully and joyously live at least another 30 years. Many of my future goals include travel with my husband and expanding my/our families of choice. However, two specific goals I now have include: 1) working fulltime as a university professor in the area of educational leadership at a prestigious university on the west coast, and 2) becoming a certified medium through the completion of Doreen Virtue's mediumship course.

The first goal was chosen because I have been employed with my current university in Arizona for more than eight years and have been teaching, primarily, undergraduate elementary education courses to pre-service teachers. While this has been extremely fulfilling and rewarding, I am interested in working again with graduate level education students. Another dream of mine has been to live near the ocean. I have lived in Arizona for over 34 years and I am ready for a change of scenery. If and when I do get hired for this new position for which I have already applied, it would require selling our home here in Arizona and moving to the west coast. My husband would pursue another job similar to the one he now has or possibly become a plant buyer which is a job he has done before and greatly enjoyed. The positive affirmations I am using to assist in bringing about this change in my and our lives are: "The perfect job at this west coast university (or an even better job on the west coast) is looking for me, and we are being brought together now. I am hired by this west coast university (or an even better employer on the west coast) where I have unlimited potential and only good lies before me. The salary is better than I could have dreamed and my husband and I find the perfect house in which to live."

The second goal I mentioned was chosen because, ever since my brother, Steve, connected with me from the other side so very soon after his death (before I was told on the earth plane), I have known that I have the ability to connect with those who have passed to the other side. I connect with my brother and my deceased aunt who were/are so special to me. I have also been able to connect with my husband's grandfather, grandmother, and father who have all passed. And, since the passing of my Grandmother Abbott in the early 1980s, I have "felt" her presence around me continuing to this day. Melissa, the leader of the Cosmic Travels Healing and Meditation Group that I attend, has told me a few times that she believes mediumship is a skill I should pursue and recommended Doreen Virtue's mediumship course. I would love to take and complete this course and become a certified medium under Doreen's mentorship. The positive affirmations I am using to assist in bringing about this change in my life are: "I have the self-esteem, power, and confidence to move forward in life with ease to become a credentialed medium. It is safe for me to become a medium with the purpose of helping others."

FINAL THOUGHTS ON HOW I KEEP SCHIZOPHRENIA AND DEPRESSION AWAY

A few people who know of my story of overcoming schizophrenia and depression have asked, "Do you have a fear of schizophrenia ever coming back into your life?" Others have asked, "What do you do to keep it away?" and "Where does your guidance come from that gives you the confidence and strength to know that it will never return?" These are all wonderful questions. I truly do not fear that I might ever have schizophrenia again. For some reason, I feel that all of the effort and work I have put into making it go away has somehow protected me from its return. Each day, I imagine a cocoon of white, gold, green, and amethyst light surrounding me with only positive energy. I call in Archangel Michael and his Band of Warriors to protect me from all harm and negativity. Each Sunday evening, I make it a practice to do an angel card reading on myself. I have all 17 of Doreen Virtue's oracle card decks and I have listed them all in the references and recommended reading section of the book. I am usually led to pull about five or six different decks of cards and ask a question such as, "What messages do the angels have for me?" or "What do I need to be working on in my life?" I shuffle the cards and one either "pops out" or I have a feeling of when to stop shuffling and I lay out a few cards from each of the decks. I look for themes and patterns and usually always see one. Typical themes that emerge have to do with forgiving myself and others, taking time to retreat, meditate, or go on a vacation, or taking better care of my health by getting rest and eating healthfully.

I also regularly take time to count my blessings and list everything I can think of to be thankful for. Additionally, I reflect on the many gifts I have been blessed with over the course of my life. Before moving on to the Reader's Workbook section of this chapter, I would like to present a synthesis or summary of the top ten gifts for which I am thankful right now in my life:

TOP TEN GIFTS

1. My husband, Scott Stackhouse
2. My mother, Helen Duke
3. My brother, Steve Duke
4. Reading books that offer new and different perspectives
5. Cosmic Travels Meditation and Healing Group
6. Hiking at the family cabin
7. Working as a university professor
8. Paying attention to my health and nutrition
9. My angels and guides
10. My friends, Jackie Earnhart, Mary Ann Schumacher, Mary Krening, and Toni Rantala

READER'S WORKBOOK: GRATITUDE LIST, GOAL-SETTING, AND POSITIVE AFFIRMATION WRITING PRACTICE TO ACHIEVE GOALS

Take a few moments now to review the gifts you listed for yourself earlier in this book and the list you created of things to be grateful or thankful for. Today, in this moment, write a new gratitude list that includes the most relevant and important gifts and things to be grateful for that are on your mind right now:

GRATITUDE LIST

1. _____

   _____

2. _____

   _____

3. _____

   _____

4. _____

   _____

5. _____

   _____

6. _____

   _____

7. _____

   _____

8. _____

_____

9. _____

_____

10. _____

_____

Next, take a look at what you wrote earlier in this book regarding your authentic self, your spiritual beliefs, and what you believe is your life's purpose. Compare your life's purpose with your new gratitude list and see if there is any overlap or connection. Write about any connections you see:

_____

_____

_____

_____

_____

_____

_____

_____

_____

_____

_____

_____

_____

_____

Now, review the answers you provided regarding plans you made to improve specific areas of your life. Take time to review 1) those areas for improvement you previously identified, 2) your new gratitude list, and 3) your life purpose. It is alright if all of the ideas are not in perfect alignment. The purpose is to get you thinking so that you can focus on a current goal you may have that you would like to achieve in the near future for which you can write a positive affirmation.

GOAL

Write a goal you have for yourself in any facet of your life. Explain why this goal is important to you and provide some ideas for how you might accomplish this goal:

_____

_____

_____

_____

_____

_____

_____

_____

_____

_____

_____

POSITIVE AFFIRMATION WRITING PRACTICE

Please review the various examples of positive affirmations I have provided in this chapter. Louise Hay, in her book *I Can Do It,* explains "It is important for you to always say your affirmations in the present tense, and without contractions. For example, typical affirmations would start: 'I have...' or 'I am...' If you say, 'I am going to...' or 'I will have...' then your thought stays out there in the future. The Universe takes your thoughts and words very literally and gives you what you say you want." Write one or more positive affirmations to support the realization and manifestation of the goal you wrote:

_____

_____

_____

_____

_____

_____

_____

_____

_____

_____

_____

_____

_____

I want to end the final chapter of this book by offering my very good wishes to you, the reader, in manifesting your goals and creating a more joyous and fulfilling life for yourself and others. I also want to remind the reader to keep working hard to maintain balance in your life and stay positive!

AFTERWORD

The story you have read is a true life, autobiographical account of my experiences with the psychological disorders of depression and schizophrenia including the development of the illnesses, possible causes, diagnoses and treatments, and ultimate recovery and maintenance of well-being through the utilization of effective strategies to become fully free of the disorders and their medications. Some of the strategies I have used are uniquely original while others should be considered modified strategies built on already published tried and true methods by many individuals referenced throughout the text and in the references and recommended reading list included at the end of this book. All of the information and strategies provided in this book are offered to those who suffer from schizophrenia, depression, and other mental illnesses and to their families, friends, and health care practitioners so all of your lives can be more joyous, purposeful, and fulfilling.

Because schizophrenia, especially, presents itself in many different forms in terms of symptoms and severity, the information I presented may not work for all schizophrenics. As I explained, my symptoms were mild and I had awareness and insight into the disorder. As mentioned previously in the book, according to the National Alliance on Mental Illness (NAMI), "research studies have shown that over 50% of those living with schizophrenia do not believe themselves to be ill. This lack of awareness or insight is known as *anosognosia*."

I believe that my experience with schizophrenia was provided as an opportunity to heal and grow and create a life that has turned out better than I might have ever imagined. Overcoming the illness of schizophrenia, for me, has proven to be both positive and transformative. However, before an individual who suffers from schizophrenia can think and live in a new and positive way leading to happiness, wholeness, and a balanced life, the mind must be recaptured and healed and the person with schizophrenia must have awareness and insight into the disorder. This journey toward wholeness can take years, but I believe it is a journey well worth taking. The journey is non-linear, complex, and multi-faceted. It requires hard work, changed thinking, healing therapies, daily practice, and continued learning.

I hope that the information I have shared about my journey to conquer schizophrenia and lead a happy and well balanced life has offered the reader a story that he or she can relate to, learn from, and/or be inspired by. I especially wanted to emphasize within this book the need to work, as a society, towards the goal of eliminating the stigma attached to any mental illness labels. There is a critical need, today, especially in light of the recent and continuing horrifying news of mass killings by people such as Jared Loughner and James Holmes who have both been diagnosed with mental illness, for the widespread development of the personal and societal attributes of compassion, understanding, and non-judgment. I, again, want to stress the importance of identifying those individuals suffering from mental illness right away and providing treatment, counseling, goal setting, education, etc. in order to prevent future violence and killing by those who are severely mentally ill and to support them so that they may, as I mentioned above, become healed, whole, and happy.

My sincerest hopes, blessings, and love to you all, including consumers (those with mental illness), along with family, friends, and caregivers of those who suffer from mental illness, in conquering schizophrenia, depression, or any other illness and finding joy and happiness in your lives. For those of you who have either already conquered an illness, assisted another in conquering illness, or will be successful in the future in overcoming schizophrenia or depression (or any other illness really), the test will be if you have been able to forget altogether that you or the person you cared for ever suffered from it. The days, weeks, months, and even years that follow during which you have totally forgotten about the illness you or a loved one once had will become true gifts for your souls to treasure!

APPENDIX: RESOURCES AND SUPPORT

Note: The phone numbers, websites, addresses, and contact information listed in this section were current as of the publication date of the book. All websites have additional resources, support groups, research publications, etc.

The National Alliance on Mental Illness (NAMI)
(*Note:* The information below is taken from the NAMI website.)

Address: 3803 N. Fairfax Drive, Suite 100, Arlington, VA 22203
Primary Phone: (703) 524-7600 Fax: (703) 524-9094
Member Services: (888) 999-6264 Helpline: (800) 950-6264
Website: www.nami.org/

State Affiliates of NAMI
(*Note:* The information below is taken from the NAMI website.)

State: ALABAMA   State Organization: NAMI Alabama
Address: 1401 I-85 Parkway Suite A, Montgomery, AL 36106-2861
Primary Phone: (334) 396-4797   Alternate Phone: (800) 626-4199
Fax: (334) 396-4794
Email Address: wlaird@namialabama.org Website: www.namialabama.org
President: James Walsh Executive Director: Wanda Laird

State: ALASKA   State Organization: NAMI Alaska
Address: 144 W. 15th Ave., Anchorage, AK 99501-5106
Primary Phone: (907) 277-1300 Alternate Phone: (800) 478-4462
Fax: (907) 277-1400
Email Address: info@nami-alaska.org Website: www.nami.org/sites/alaska

President: Scott Owens

State: ARIZONA   State Organization: NAMI Arizona
  Address: 5025 E. Washington St., Suite 112, Phoenix, AZ 85034
  Primary Phone: (602) 244-8166 Alternate Phone: (800) 626-5022
  Fax: (602) 252-1349
  Email Address: namiaz@namiaz.org Website: www.namiaz.org
  President: David Covington

State: ARKANSAS   State Organization: NAMI Arkansas
  Address: 1012 Autumn Rd., Suite 1, Little Rock, AR 72211-3704
  Primary Phone: (501) 661-1548 Alternate Phone: (800) 844-0381
  Fax: (501) 664-0264
  Email Address: nami-ar@namiarkansas.org Website: www.namiarkansas.org
  Executive Director: Kim Arnold

State: CALIFORNIA   State Organization: NAMI California
  Address: 1851 Heritage Lane, Suite 150, Sacramento, CA 95815
  Primary Phone: (916) 567-0163 Fax: (916) 567-1757
  Email Address: nami.california@namicalifornia.org
  Website: www.namicalifornia.org
  President: Dorothy Hendrickson Executive Director: Jessica Cruz

State: COLORADO   State Organization: NAMI Colorado
  Address: 1100 Fillmore St., Suite 201, Denver, CO 80206-3334
  Primary Phone: (303) 321-3104 Alternate Phone: (888) 566-6264
  Fax: (303) 321-0912
  Email Address: admin@namicolorado.org Website: www.namicolorado.org
  President: Greg Coleman Executive Director: Scott Glaser
  Additional Contact: Liz Parker

State: CONNECTICUT   State Organization: NAMI Connecticut
  Address: 241 Main St., 5th Floor, Hartford, CT 06106-1862
  Primary Phone: (860) 882-0236 Alternate Phone: (800) 215-3021
  Fax: (860) 882-0240
  Email Address: namicted@namict.org Website: www.namict.org
  President: Robert Davidson Executive Director: Kate Mattias

State: DELAWARE   State Organization: NAMI Delaware
  Address: 2400 W. 4th St., Wilmington, DE 19805-3306
  Primary Phone: (302) 427-0787 Alternate Phone: (888) 427-2075
  Email Address: namide@namide.org Website: www.namide.org
  President: Mary Berger Executive Director: Matt Stehl

State: FLORIDA   State Organization: NAMI Florida
  Address: 1030 E. Lafayette St., Suite 10, Tallahassee, FL 32301-4587
  Primary Phone: (877) 626-4352 Alternate Phone: (850) 671-4445
  Fax: (850) -671-5272
  Email Address: info@namiflorida.org Website: www.namiflorida.org

President: James Sleeper Executive Director: Judith Evans
Additional Contact: Carol Weber

State: GEORGIA   State Organization: NAMI Georgia
Address: 3050 Presidential Drive, Suite 202, Atlanta, GA 30340-3916
Primary Phone: (770) 234-0855 Alternate Phone: (800) 728-1052
Fax: (770) 234-0237
Email Address: namigoergia@namiga.org Website: www.namiga.org
President: Bill Kissel Additional Contact: Eric Spencer

State: HAWAII   State Organization: NAMI Hawaii State
Address: 770 Kapiolani Blvd., Suite 613, Honolulu, HI 96813-5212
Primary Phone: (808) 591-1208 Fax: (808) 591-2058
Email Address: info@namihawaii.org Website: www.namihawaii.org
President: Ann Collins Executive Director: Kathleen Hasegawa

State: IDAHO   State Organization: NAMI Idaho
Address: 4097 Bottle Bay Rd., Sagle, ID 83860-9009
Primary Phone: (208) 242-7430
Email Address: namiidaho@yahoo.com Website: www.nami.org/sites/namiidaho
President: Douglas McKnight Executive Director: Zina Magee

State: ILLINOIS   State Organization: NAMI Illinois
Address: 218 W. Lawrence Ave., Springfield, IL 62704-2612
Primary Phone: (217) 522-1403 Alternate Phone: (800) 346-4572
Fax: (217) 522-3598
Email Address: namiil@sbcglobal.net Website: www.il.nami.org
President: Hug Brady Executive Director: Lora Thomas

State: INDIANA   State Organization: NAMI Indiana
Address: P. O. Box 22697, Indianapolis, IN 46222-0697
Primary Phone: (317) 925-9399 Alternate Phone: (800) 677-6442
Fax: (317) 925-9398
Email Address: info@namiindiana.org Website: www.namiindiana.org
President: Harriet Rosen Executive Director: Pamela McConey

State: IOWA   State Organization: NAMI Iowa
Address: ATTN: Nancy Hale, 5911 Meredith Dr., Ste E, Des Moines, IL 50322-1903
Primary Phone: (515) 254-0417 Alternate Phone: (800) 417-0417
Fax: (515) 254-1103
Email Address: info@namiiowa.com Website: www.namiiowa.com
President: Diane Banasiak Executive Director: Nancy Hale

State: KANSAS   State Organization: NAMI Kansas
Address: 610 SW 10th Ave., Suite 203, Topeka, KS 66612-1673
Primary Phone: (785) 233-0755 Alternate Phone: (800) 539-2660
Fax: (785) 233-4804
Email Address: info@namikansas.org Website: www.namikansas.org
President: John Brennan Executive Director: Richard Cagan

State: KENTUCKY   State Organization: NAMI Kentucky
Address: c/o Sommerset Community College, 808 Monticito St., Somerset, KY 42501-2973
Primary Phone: (606) 451-6935 Alternate Phone: (800) 257-5081
Email Address: namiky@bellsouth.net
Website: www.nami.org/MSTemplate.cfm?micrositeID=157
President: Wendy Morris Executive Director: Cathy Epperson

State: LOUISIANA   State Organization: NAMI Louisiana
Address: P. O. Box 40517, Baton Rouge, LA 70835-0517
Primary Phone: (225) 291-6262 Alternate Phone: (866) 851-6264
Fax: (225) 291-6244
Email Address: info@namilouisiana.org Website: www.namilouisiana.org
President: Stephanie Boyd Executive Director: Jennifer Jantz

State: MAINE   State Organization: NAMI Maine
Address: 1 Bangor St.,Augusta, ME 04330-4701
Primary Phone: (207) 622-5767 Alternate Phone: (800) 464-5767
Fax: (207) 621-8430
Email Address: info@namimaine.org Website: www.namimaine.org
President: Marcia Homestead Executive Director: Carol Carothers

State: MARYLAND   State Organization: NAMI Maryland
Address: 10630 Little Patuxent Parkway, Suite 475, Columbia, MD 21044-3264
Primary Phone: (410) 884-8691 Alternate Phone: (877) 878-2371
Fax: (410) 884-8695
Email Address: info@namimd.org Website: www.namimd.org
President: Don Slater Executive Director: Kate Farinholt

State: MASSACHUSETTS   State Organization: NAMI Massachusetts
Address: 400 West Cummings Park, Suite 6650, Woburn, MA 01801-6528
Primary Phone: (781) 938-4048 Alternate Phone: (800) 370-9085
Fax: (781)-938-4069
Email Address: info@namimass.org Website: www.namimass.org
President: Guy Beales Executive Director: Laurie Martinelli

State: MICHIGAN   State Organization: NAMI Michigan
Address: 921 N. Washington Ave., Lansing, MI 48906-5137
Primary Phone: (517) 485-4049 Alternate Phone: (800) 331-4264
Fax: (517) 485-2333
Email Address: info@namimi.org Website: www.namimi.org
President: David Ballenberger Executive Director: Linda Burghardt

State: MINNESOTA   State Organization: NAMI Minnesota
Address: 800 Transfer Rd., Suite 31, Saint Paul, MN 55114-1414
Primary Phone: (651) 645-2948 Alternate Phone: 1(888) NAMI-HELPS
Fax: (651) 645-7379
Email Address: namihelps@namimn.org Website: www.namihelps.org
President: William Bond Executive Director: Sue Abderholden

State: MISSISSIPPI   State Organization: NAMI Mississippi
   Address: 411 Briarwood Dr., Suite 401, Jackson, MS 39206-3058
   Primary Phone: (601) 899-9058 Alternate Phone: (800) 357-0388
   Fax: (601) 956-6380
   Email Address: stateoffice@namims.org Website: www.namims.org
   President: W. Wes Johnson Executive Director: Tonya Tate

State: MISSOURI   State Organization: NAMI Missouri
   Address: 3405 West Truman Blvd., Suite 102, Jefferson City, MO 65109-2501
   Primary Phone: (573) 634-7727 Alternate Phone: (800) 374-2138
   Fax: (573) 761-5636
   Email Address: namimofamilies@yahoo.com Website: www.nami.org/sites/MO
   President: Tim Harlan Executive Director: Cindi Keele

State: MONTANA   State Organization: NAMI Montana
   Address: P. O. Box 1021, 616 Helena Ave., Suite 218, Helena, MT 59624-1021
   Primary Phone: (406) 443-7871 Fax: (406) 862-6357
   Email Address: info@namimt.org Website: www.namimt.org
   President: Gary Popiel Executive Director: Matthew Kuntz

State: NEBRASKA   State Organization: NAMI Nebraska
   Address: 415 S. 25th Ave., Bldg. LH, Omaha, NE 68131-3654
   Primary Phone: (402) 345-8101 Alternate Phone: (877) 463-6264
   Fax: (402) 346-4070
   Email Address: tadams@naminebraska.org Website: www.nami.org/sites/ne
   President: Timothy Cuddigan Executive Director: Tom Adams

State: NEVADA   State Organization: NAMI Nevada
   Address: 1170 Curti Dr., Reno, NV 89502
   Primary Phone: (775) 329-3260 Alternate Phone: (775) 688-3317
   Fax: (775) 329-1618
   Email Address: jtyler@nnamhs.state.nv.us
   President: Joe Tyler

State: NEW HAMPSHIRE   State Organization: NAMI New Hampshire
   Address: 15 Green St., Concord, NH 03301-4020
   Primary Phone: (603) 225-5359 Alternate Phone: (800) 242-6264
   Fax: (603) 228-8848
   Email Address: info@naminh.org Website: www.naminh.org
   President: Jonathan Routhier Executive Director: Kenneth Norton

State: NEW JERSEY   State Organization: NAMI New Jersey
   Address: 1562 US Highway 130, New Brunswick, NJ 08902-3004
   Primary Phone: (732) 940-0991 Fax: (732) 940-0355
   Email Address: info@naminj.org Website: www.naminj.org
   President: Mark Perrin Executive Director: Sylvia Axelrod

State: NEW MEXICO   State Organization: NAMI New Mexico
   Address: 8015 Mountain Road Pl., NE, Ste. 101, Albuquerque, NM 87110

Primary Phone: (505) 260-0154 Fax: (505) 260-0342
Email Address: naminm@aol.com Website: www.nm.nami.org
President: Kris Ericson Executive Director: Kim Ahiborn

State: NEW YORK   State Organization: NAMI New York State
Address: 260 Washington Ave., Albany, NY 12210-1312
Primary Phone: (518) 462-2000 Alternate Phone: (800) 950-3228
Fax: (518) 462-3811
Email Address: info@naminys.org Website: www.naminys.org
President: Sherry Grenz Executive Director: Donald Capone

State: NORTH CAROLINA   State Organization: NAMI North Carolina
Address: 309 W. Millbrook Rd., Ste. 121, Charlotte, NC 27609-4394
Primary Phone: (919) 788-0801 Alternate Phone: (800) 451-9682
Fax: (919) 788-0906
Email Address: mail@naminc.org Website: www.naminc.org
President: David Bullins Executive Director: Debra Dihoff

State: NORTH DAKOTA   State Organization: NAMI North Dakota
Address: 4068 Acorn Ct., Grand Forks, ND 58201-7157
Primary Phone: (701) 757-0282
Email Address: naminorthdakota@gmail.com Website: www.namind.org
President: Barb Dahlen

State: OHIO   State Organization: NAMI Ohio
Address: 747 East Broad St., Columbus, OH 43205
Primary Phone: (614) 224-2700 Alternate Phone: (800) 686-2646
Fax: (614) 224-5400
Email Address: namiohio@namiohio.org Website: www.namiohio.org
President: Senator Robert Spada Executive Director: Terry Russell

State: OKLAHOMA   State Organization: NAMI Oklahoma
Address: 4200 Perimeter Center Dr., Ste. 150, Oklahoma City, OK 73112
Primary Phone: (405) 230-1900 Alternate Phone: (800) 583-1264
Fax: (405) 230-1903
Email Address: namiok@coxinet.net Website: www.ok.nami.org
President: Paula Walker Executive Director: David Gordon

State: OREGON   State Organization: NAMI Oregon
Address: 4701 SE 24th Ave., Ste. E, Portland, OR 97202-4783
Primary Phone: (503) 230-8009 Alternate Phone: (800) 343-6264
Fax: (503) 230-2751
Email Address: namioregon@namior.org Website: www.nami.org/sites/NAMIoregon
President: Kim Schneiderman Executive Director: Christopher Bouneff
Additional Contact: Michelle Madison Additional Contact: Peter Link

State: PENNSYLVANIA   State Organization: NAMI Pennsylvania
Address: 2149 North 2nd St., Harrisburg, PA 17110-1005
Primary Phone: (717) 238-1514 Alternate Phone: (800) 223-0500

Fax: (717) 238-4390
Email Address: nami-pa@nami-pa.org Website: www.namipa.nami.org
President: Suzanna Vogel-Scibilia Executive Director: James Jordan

State: RHODE ISLAND   State Organization: NAMI Rhode Island
Address: 154 Waterman St., Ste. 5B, Providence, RI 02906-3116
Primary Phone: (401) 331-3060 Alternate Phone: (800) 749-3197
Fax: (401) 274-3020
Email Address: chaznami@cox.net Website: www.namirhodeisland.org
President: Marcia Boyd Executive Director: Charles Gross

State: SOUTH CAROLINA   State Organization: NAMI South Carolina
Address: P. O. Box 1267, 5000 Thurmond Mall Blvd., Columbia, SC 29202-1267
Primary Phone: (800) 788-5131 Alternate Phone: (803) 733-9592
Fax: (803) 733-9593
Email Address: namisc@namisc.org Website: www.namisc.org
President: Joan Herbert Executive Director: Bill Lindsey

State: SOUTH DAKOTA   State Organization: NAMI South Dakota
Address: P. O. Box 88808, Sioux Falls, SD 57109-8808
Primary Phone: (605) 271-1871 Alternate Phone: (800) 551-2531
Fax: (605) 271-1871
Email   Address: namisd@midconetwork.com   Website: www.nami.org/sites/
NAMISouthDakota
President: Ken Heeren Executive Director: Phyllis Arends

State: TENNESSEE   State Organization: NAMI Tennessee
Address: 1101 Kermit Dr., Ste. 605, Nashville, TN 37217-2126
Primary Phone: (615) 361-6608 Alternate Phone: (800) 467-3589
Fax: (615) 361-6698
Email Address: info@namitn.org Website: www.namitn.org
President: Richard Baxter Executive Director: Roger Stewart
Additional Contact: Brenda Stacey-Scott

State: TEXAS   State Organization: NAMI Texas
Address: Fountain Park Plaza III, 2000 South IH35, Ste. 140, Austin, TX 78704
Primary Phone: (800) 633-3760 Alternate Phone: (512) 693-2000
Fax: (512) 693-8000
Email Address: kjeschke@namitexas.org Website: www.namitexas.org
President: Andrea Hazlitt Executive Director: Robin Peyson

State: UTAH   State Organization: NAMI Utah
Address: 1600 West 2000 South, Ste. 202, West Valley City, UT 84121
Primary Phone: (801) 323-9900 Fax: (801) 323-9799
Email Address: education@namiut.org Website: www.namiut.org
President: Zara Juillerat Executive Director: Rebecca Glathar

State: VERMONT   State Organization: NAMI Vermont
Address: 162 South Main St., Waterbury, VT 05676-1519

Primary Phone: (802) 244-1396 Alternate Phone: (800) 639-6480
Fax: (802) 244-1405
Email Address: info@namivt.org Website: www.namivt.org
President: Judy Rosenstreich Executive Director: Wendy Beinner
Additional Contact: Linda Anderson

State: VIRGINIA   State Organization: NAMI Virginia
Address: P. O. Box 8260, Richmond, VA 23226-0260
Primary Phone: (804) 285-8264 Alternate Phone: (888) 486-8264
Fax: (804) 285-8264
Email Address: namiva@comcast.net Website: www.namivirginia.org
President: Bob Williams Executive Director: Mira Signer

State: WASHINGTON   State Organization: NAMI Washington
Address: 7500 Greenwood Ave. N, Seattle, WA 98103
Primary Phone: (206) 783-4288 Fax: (206) 783-4614
Email Address: office@namiwa.org Website: www.namiwa.org
President: Farrell Adrian

State: WEST VIRGINIA   State Organization: NAMI West Virginia
(further local West Virginia affiliates can be found on NAMI website: www.nami.org/)

State: WISCONSIN   State Organization: NAMI Wisconsin
Address: 4233 W. Beltline Hwy., Madison, WI 53711-3814
Primary Phone: (608) 268-6000 Alternate Phone: (800) 236-2988
Fax: (608) 268-6004
Email Address: nami@namiwisconsin.org Website: www.namiwisconsin.org
President: Sandy Hall Executive Director: Julianne Carbin
Additional Contact: Patti Jo Severson

State: WYOMING   State Organization: NAMI Wyoming
Address: 133 W. 6th St., Casper, WY 82601-3124
Primary Phone: (307) 264-2573 Alternate Phone: (888) 882-4968
Fax: (307) 265-0968
Email Address: nami-wyo@qwestoffice.net Website: www.namiwyoming.org
President: Deion Hagemeister Executive Director: Andrea Hammond
Additional Contact: Jane Johnson

NAMI Education, Training, and Peer Support
(*Note:* The information below is taken from the NAMI website)

NAMI Family-to-Family

Website: www.nami.org/f2f

Course description: For family members, partners, and friends of someone living with a mental illness. (12-week course)

Course review: "Before I took the course, I felt along and overwhelmed dealing with my daughter's mental illness. By taking this course, I have met others who are going through the same things I am and have learned about many resources that I never knew existed."

NAMI Peer-to-Peer

Website: www.nami.org/peertopeer

Course description: For consumers (people living with a mental illness) (10-week course)

Course review: "Peer-to-Peer has allowed me to take the focus off my illness and learn to balance it with the rest of my life. By engaging in recovery I am able to be more relaxed and productive both at work and home."

NAMI Basics

Website: www.nami.org/basics

Course description: For parents and other caregivers of children and adolescents living with mental illness. (Meets once a week for six weeks or twice a week for three weeks)

Course review: "This is the best program for families with children. It answers so many questions for parents. It can change and improve so many lives."

NAMI Provider Education Website: www.nami.org/providereducation

Course description:	For providers of mental health services. (Meets for six weeks)
Course review:	"This course has given me a much greater appreciation for the heroism of people living with mental illness and for the families who love and support them."

NAMI Parents and Teachers as Allies

Website: www.nami.org/template.cfm?section=Schools_and_Education

Course description:	For school professionals. (Two hour in-service program)
Course review:	"This program gave me a new understanding of the importance of my role in early recognition of kids with symptoms of mental illness and the urgency of early intervention on their behalf."

NAMI Connection Website: www.nami.org/connection

Course description:	For consumers. (Meets once a week)
Course review:	"I am not alone! There is a place where people understand me, are there to help me, and I feel better about myself when I help someone else. I can get involved in NAMI Connection and make a difference!"

NAMI Family Support Group

Support group description:	For family members and/or loved ones of someone living with a mental illness. (Meets once a month)
Support group review:	"Using the support group model is so essential to the success of our family support groups. Without the training, networking, and support of the group members, I fear that support groups would become nothing more than 'cry' sessions or 'gripe' sessions. As a group, the collective wisdom covered a lot of possibilities towards the issues."

NAMI In Our Own Voice Website: www.nami.org/ioov

Presentation description: For the general public. (Recurring one time presentations)

Presentation review: "The reason why this program is such a valuable resource for us is that it puts a human face on people who are living successfully with a mental illness."

NAMI Hearts and Minds Website: www.nami.org/heartsandminds

Course description: For the general public (Online, interactive, educational initiative)

Course description: "This course has literally been a life saver. It has opened my eyes to better understanding my illness and methods of recovery I did not know about before taking the course."

Weight Loss

Weight Watchers   website: www.WeightWatchers.com

REFERENCES AND RECOMMENDED READING

Baha'u'llah, The Bab, & 'Abdu'l-Baha. (1979). *Bahai prayers: A selection of the prayers revealed by Baha'u'llah, The Bab, and 'Abdu'l-Baha.* Wilmette, IL: Bahai Publishing Trust.

Battie, S. (2006). *Channelling: Use your psychic powers to contact your spirit guides.* London: Godsfield Press, A Division of Octopus Publishing Group LTD.

Bloomfield, H. (1998). *Healing anxiety with herbs.* New York: Harper Collins Publishers, Inc.

Brinkman, R., & Kirschner, R. (2002). *Dealing with people you can't stand.* New York: McGraw-Hill.

Brinkman, R., & Kirschner, R. (2003). *Who do you think you are anyway?* New York: McGraw-Hill.

Browne, S. (2006). *Exploring the levels of creation.* Carlsbad, CA: Hay House, Inc.

Browne, S. (2000). *God, creation, and tools for life.* Carlsbad, CA: Hay House, Inc.

Browne, S. (2006). *If you could see what I see.* Carlsbad, CA: Hay House, Inc.

Browne, S., & Harrison, L. (2005). *Phenomenon: Everything you need to know about the paranormal.* New York: Dutton, Published by Penguin Group.

Browne, S., & Harrison, L. (2005). *Prophecy: What the future holds for you.* New York: New American Library, A Division of Penguin Group.

Browne, S., & Harrison, L. (2007). *Psychic children: Revealing the intuitive gifts and hidden abilities of boys and girls.* New York: Dutton, Published by Penguin Group.

Browne, S. (2009). *Psychic healing: Using the tools of a medium to cure whatever ails you.* Carlsbad, CA: Hay House, Inc.

Browne, S. (2007). *Secret societies and how they affect our lives today.* Carlsbad, CA: Hay House, Inc.

Browne, S. (2007). *Spiritual connections: How to find spirituality throughout all the relationships in your life.* Carlsbad, CA: Hay House, Inc.

Browne, S. (2009). *Sylvia Browne: Accepting the psychic torch.* Carlsbad, CA: Hay House, Inc.

Browne, S., & Harrison, L. (2002). *Sylvia Browne's book of dreams.* Carlsbad, CA: Hay House, Inc.

Browne, S. (2008). *Temples on the other side: How wisdom from "beyond the veil" can help you right now.* Carlsbad, CA: Hay House, Inc.

Burns, B. (1992). *Channelling: Evolutionary exercises for channels* (Vywamus channeled by Barbara Burns). Sedona, AZ: Light Technology Publishing.

Carper, J. (2000). *Your miracle brain.* New York: Harper Collins Publishers, Inc.

Carter, R. (1998). *Helping someone with mental illness.* New York: Random House.

Castaneda, C. (1978). *The teachings of Don Juan: A Yaqui way of knowledge.* Penguin Books.

Chapman, G. (2010). *The 5 love languages (men's edition): The secret to love that lasts.*

Chicago, IL: Northfield Publishing.

Chapman, G. (2007). *The heart of the five love languages.* Chicago, IL: Northfield Publishing.

Choquette, S. (2004). *Trust your vibes.* Carlsbad, CA: Hay House, Inc.

Choquette, S. (1997). *Your heart's desire.* New York: Three Rivers Press.

Collins, T. (2001). *Feng shui personal paradise cards*. Carlsbad, CA: Hay House, Inc.

Cortens, T., & Shaman, W. (1997). *The angels' script*. Oxfordshire: CAER SIDI Publications.

Dass, R. (1971). *Be here now*. Hanuman Foundation Publishers.

Dass, R. (2000). *Still here: Embracing aging, changing, and dying*. New York: Riverhead Books, A Division of Penguin Putnam Inc.

Dean, A. (1986). *Night light: A book of nighttime meditations*. San Francisco: Harper & Row, Publishers.

Dean, A. (2000). *Pleasant dreams: Nighttime meditations for peace of mind*. Carlsbad, CA: Hay House, Inc.

Dyer, W. (2009). *Excuses begone! How to change lifelong, self-defeating thinking habits*. Carlsbad, CA: Hay House, Inc.

Dyer, W. (2003). *Getting in the gap: Making conscious contact with god through meditation*. Carlsbad, CA: Hay House, Inc.

Dyer, W. (2001). *Ten secrets for success and inner peace*. Carlsbad, CA: Hay House, Inc.

Dyer, W. (2004). *The power of intention: Learning to co-create your world your way*. Carlsbad, CA: Hay House, Inc.

Dyer, W. (2012). *Wishes fulfilled: Mastering the art of manifesting*. Carlsbad, CA: Hay House, Inc.

Emoto, M. (2004). *The hidden messages in water*. Hillsboro, OR: Beyond Words Publishing, Inc.

Garten, M. (1967). *The health secrets of a naturopathic doctor*. New York: Lancer Books.

Gibran, K. (1972). *The prophet*. New York: Alfred A. Knopf.

Gray, H. (1974). *Gray's anatomy*. Philadelphia, PA: Running Press Book Publishers.

Gray, J. (2001). *Mars Venus cards*. New York: Harper Collins.

Hay, L. (1998). *Heal your body A-Z: The mental causes for physical illness and the way to overcome them*. Carlsbad, CA: Hay House, Inc.

Hay, L. (2004). *I can do it: How to use affirmations to change your life.* Carlsbad, CA: Hay House, Inc.

Hay, L. (2000). *Inner wisdom: Meditations for the heart and soul.* Carlsbad, CA: Hay House, Inc.

Hay, L. (1999). *Power thought cards.* Carlsbad, CA: Hay House, Inc.

Hay, L. (1988). *You can heal your life.* Carlsbad, CA: Hay House, Inc.

Hicks, E., & Hicks, J. (2004). *The teachings of Abraham well-being cards.* Carlsbad, CA: Hay House, Inc.

Holmes, E. (1938). *Science of mind* (revised edition).

Johnson, S. (1998). *Who moved my cheese?* New York: G.P. Putnam's Sons.

Jones, M. (2010). *The little book of light: 111 ways to bring light into your life* (3rd ed.). Portland, OR: Radiant Being Publishing Company.

Kelly, E. (1997). *Spiritual journey: How to get through the day.* Yellow Springs, OH: Cimarron Books.

Kenyon, T., & Essene, V. (1996). *The hathor material: Messages from an ascended civilization.* Orcas, WA: ORB Communications.

Kenyon, T., & Sion, J. (2004). *The magdalen manuscript: The alchemies of Horus and the sex Magic of Isis.* Orcas, WA: ORB Communications.

Kovan, D. (2001). *Secrets of numerology.* New York: DK Publishing, Inc.

Kiyosaki, R. (1999). *Cash flow quadrant.* New York: Warner Business Books.

Kiyosaki, R. (1999). *Rich dad, poor dad.* New York: Warner Business Books.

Lampert, V. (2000). *Angel messages: A heaven-sent book and pack of 52 uniquely inspirational cards.* New York: A Bulfinch Press Book, Little, Brown and Company.

Leman, K. (2009). *The birth order book: Why you are the way you are.* Grand Rapids, MI: Revell, A Division of Baker Publishing Group.

Leman, K. (2008). *Sheet music: Uncovering the secrets of sexual intimacy in marriage.* Carol Stream, IL: Tyndale House Publishers, Inc.

LeMay, K. (2009). *The generosity plan: Sharing your time, treasure, and talent to shape the world*. New York: Atria Books: A Division of Simon and Schuster.

Love, P., & Stosny, S. (2007). *How to improve your marriage without talking about it*. New York: Broadway Books.

MacLaine, S. (2007). *Sage-ing while age-ing*. New York: Atria Books, A Division of Simon and Schuster, Inc.

Marohn, S. (2003). *The natural guide to schizophrenia*. Charlottesville, VA: Hampton Roads Publishing Company, Inc.

McGraw, P. (2008). *Real life: Preparing for the 7 most challenging days of your life*. New York: Free Press.

McGraw, P. (2001). *Self matters*. New York: Simon and Schuster.

McLaren, K. (2010). *Emotional vitality: 5 empathic skills to awaken your natural intelligence*. Boulder, CO: Sounds True.

McLaren, K. (2010). *The language of emotions. What your feelings are trying to tell you*. Boulder, CO: Sounds True.

McMahon, S. (1992). *The portable therapist: Wise and inspiring answers to the questions, people in therapy ask most*. New York: A Dell Trade Paperback.

Mehl-Madrona, L. (1997). *Coyote medicine*. New York: Scribner.

Mehl-Madrona, L. (2011). *Healing with spirit: Native American stories, insights, and guided practices*. Boulder, CO: Sounds True.

Miguel Ruiz, D. (1997). *The four agreements: Toltec wisdom cards*. San Rafael, CA: Amber-Allen Publishing.

Myss, C. (2003). *Archetype cards*. Carlsbad, CA: Hay House, Inc.

Myss, C. (2007). *Entering the castle: An inner path to god and your soul*. New York: Free Press, A Division of Simon and Schuster, Inc.

Myss, C. (2004). *Essential guide for healers*. Boulder, CO: Sounds True.

Myss, C. (2003). *Fundamentals of spiritual alchemy: Live workshop*. Carlsbad, CA: Hay House Audio.

Myss, C. (2002). *Self-esteem: Your fundamental power*. Boulder, CO: Sounds True.

Myss, C. (2007). *The mysterious will of divinity*. Boulder, CO: Sounds True.

Myss, C. (2011). *The power of prayer: Guidance, prayers, and wisdom for listening to the divine*. Boulder, CO: Sounds True.

NAMI (National Alliance on Mental Illness). (2012). Website: www.nami. org/

Ness, C. (2001). *Secrets of dreams*. New York: DK Publishing, Inc.

Northrup, C. (2006). *The wisdom of menopause: Creating physical and emotional health during the change*. New York: Bantam Dell, A Division of Random House, Inc.

Orloff, J. (2006). *Positive energy practices: How to attract uplifting people and combat energy vampires*. Boulder, CO: Sounds True.

Prophet, E. (1997). *Violet frame to heal body, mind, and soul*. Corwin Springs, MT: Summit University Press.

Quan Yin, A. (1996). *The Pleiadian workbook: Awakening your divine ka*. Rochester, VT: Bear and Company.

Ramacharaka, Y. (1909). *The Hindu yogi practical water cure*. Chicago, IL: The Yoga Publication Society.

Randall-May, C. (2010). *Healing and the creative response: Four key steps shared by healers and artists*. CayMay Press.

Randall-May, C. (2005). *The intuitive career: How to succeed as a consultant, reader, or healer*. CayMay Press.

Raven Clan. (June, 2005). *Raven Clan Wisdom Level Three Clearing Report*. (email).

Rohm, R. (2000). *Positive personality profiles*. Atlanta, GA: Personality Insights, Inc.

Rohm, R. (1997). *Who do you think you are anyway?* Atlanta, GA: Personality Insights, Inc.

Rosen, R. (2010). *Spirited: Connect to the guides all around you*. New York: Harper Collins Publishers.

Rosenberg, L. (2000). *Mahatma Reiki level I handbook*. (Class handout).

Royal, P. (1976). *Herbally yours: A comprehensive herbal handbook simple enough for the Herbal students, complete enough for the herbal practitioner.* Provo, UT: Microlith Printing Inc. An Amtec Subsidiary.

Sass, L. (1995). *The paradoxes of delusion: Wittgenstein, Schreber and the schizophrenic mind.* Cornell Publishing.

Schucman, H. (1996). *A course in miracles.* Mill Valley, CA: Foundation for Inner Peace.

Segal, I. (2010). *The secret language of colour cards.* Victoria, Australia: Blue Angel Publishing.

Shimoff, M. (2008). *Happy for no reason: 7 steps to being happy from the inside out.* New York: Free Press.

Shubert, C. (1999). *Develop and control your psychic ability through guided meditation and visualization* (CD). Carrie Shubert Copyright.

Shubert, C. (2002). *Living in the third dimensional soap opera: A spiritual guide to sanity.* Carrie Shubert Copyright.

Taichi-ren, T. (1999). *What is lightbody?* Lithia Springs, GA: New Leaf Distributing.

Theole, S. (1996). *The woman's book of courage: Meditations for empowerment and peace of mind.* New York: MJF Books.

Torrey, E. (2001). *Surviving schizophrenia: A manual for families, consumers, and providers.* New York: Harper Perennial Publishers.

Van Praagh, J. (2000). *Healing grief: Reclaiming life after any loss.* New York: A Dutton Book, Penguin Putnam, Inc.

Van Praagh, J. (2003). *Meditations with James Van Praagh.* New York: A Fireside Book, Simon and Schuster.

Virtue, D. (2004). *Angel medicine.* Carlsbad, CA: Hay House, Inc.

Virtue, D., & Brown, L. (2005). *Angel numbers.* Carlsbad, CA: Hay House, Inc.

Virtue, D., & Valentine, R. (2012). *Angel tarot cards.* Carlsbad, CA: Hay House, Inc.

Virtue, D. (1997). *Angel therapy.* Carlsbad, CA: Hay House, Inc.

Virtue, D. (2008). *Angel therapy oracle cards.* Carlsbad, CA: Hay House, Inc.

Virtue, D. (2004). *Archangel oracle cards.* Carlsbad, CA: Hay House, Inc.

Virtue, D. (2009). *Archangel Michael oracle cards.* Carlsbad, CA: Hay House, Inc.

Virtue, D. (2010). *Archangel Raphael healing oracle cards.* Carlsbad, CA: Hay House, Inc.

Virtue, D. (2003). *Archangels and ascended masters: A guide to working and healing with divinities and deities.* Carlsbad, CA: Hay House, Inc.

Virtue, D. (2007). *Ascended masters oracle cards.* Carlsbad, CA: Hay House, Inc.

Virtue, D. (1998). *Chakra clearing: Awakening your spiritual power to know and heal.* Carlsbad, CA: Hay House, Inc.

Virtue, D. (2006). *Daily guidance from your angels.* Carlsbad, CA: Hay House, Inc.

Virtue, D. (2006). *Daily guidance from your angels oracle cards.* Carlsbad, CA: Hay House, Inc.

Virtue, D. (2006). *Divine magic: The seven sacred secrets of manifestation (A new interpretation of the classic hermetic manual the kybalion.* Carlsbad, CA: Hay House, Inc.

Virtue, D. (2000). *Divine prescriptions: Using your sixth sense – spiritual solutions for you and your loved ones.* Carlsbad, CA: Hay House, Inc.

Virtue, D. (2002). *Earth angels: A pocket guide for incarnated angels, elementals, starpeople, walk-ins, and wizards.* Carlsbad, CA: Hay House, Inc.

Virtue, D., & Prelitz, B. (2001). *Eating in the light: Making the switch to vegetarianism on your spiritual path.* Carlsbad, CA: Hay House, Inc.

Virtue, D. (2004). *Goddess guidance oracle cards.* Carlsbad, CA: Hay House, Inc.

Virtue, D. (2005). *Goddesses and angels: Awakening your inner high-priestess and "Source-eress."* Carlsbad, CA: Hay House, Inc.

Virtue, D. (1999). *Healing with the angels oracle cards.* Carlsbad, CA: Hay House, Inc.

Virtue, D. (1999). *Healing with the angels: How the angels can assist you in every area of your life.* Carlsbad, CA: Hay House, Inc.

Virtue, D. (2001). *Healing with the fairies: Messages, manifestations, and love from the world of the fairies.* Carlsbad, CA: Hay House, Inc.

Virtue, D. (2001). *Healing with fairies oracle cards.* Carlsbad, CA: Hay House, Inc.

Virtue, D. (1996). *I'd change my life if I had more time: A practical guide to making dreams come true.* Carlsbad, CA: Hay House, Inc.

Virtue, D. (2011). *Life purpose oracle cards.* Carlsbad, CA: Hay House, Inc.

Virtue, D. (2003). *Magical mermaids and dolphins oracle cards.* Carlsbad, CA: Hay House, Inc.

Virtue, D. (2008). *Magical messages from the fairies oracle cards.* Carlsbad, CA: Hay House, Inc.

Virtue, D. (2005). *Magical unicorn oracle cards.* Carlsbad, CA: Hay House, Inc.

Virtue, D. (2002). *Messages from your angels: What your angels want you to know.* Carlsbad, CA: Hay House, Inc.

Virtue, D. (2002). *Messages from your angels: What your angels want you to know oracle cards.* Carlsbad, CA: Hay House, Inc.

Virtue, D. (2007). *Realms of the earth angels: More information for incarnated angels, elementals, wizards, and other lightworkers.* Carlsbad, CA: Hay House, Inc.

Virtue, D. (2005). *Saints and angels oracle cards.* Carlsbad, CA: Hay House, Inc.

Virtue, D. (2011). *The angel therapy handbook.* Carlsbad, CA: Hay House, Inc.

Virtue, D. (2010). *The healing miracles of archangel Raphael.* Carlsbad, CA: Hay House, Inc.

Virtue, D. (1997). *The lightworker's way: Awakening your spiritual power to know and heal.* Carlsbad, CA: Hay House, Inc.

Virtue, D. (2012). *The romance angels oracle cards.* Carlsbad, CA: Hay House, Inc.

Weil, A. (1997). *8 weeks to optimum health.* New York: Fawcett Columbine.

Weiss, B. (2002). *Mirrors of time: Using regression for physical, emotional, and spiritual healing.* Carlsbad, CA: Hay House, Inc.

Williamson, M. (2002). *Everyday grace: Having hope, finding forgiveness, and making miracles.* New York: Riverhead Books.

Wulfing, S. (2001). *Lovers oracle.* Belgium: Bluestar Communications.

Yogananda, P. (1973). *Autobiography of a yogi.* Los Angeles, CA: Self-Realization Fellowship Publishers.

Zerner, A., & Farber, M. (2008). *Little reminders: The law of attraction: 36 oracle cards to guide you to wealth and prosperity.* New York: Sterling Publishing Company.

Ziglar, Z. (1969). *Zig Ziglar's favorite quotations.* Lombard, IL: Great Quotations, Inc.

Zimmerman, L. (2011). *The sacred wisdom of the American Indians.* Duncan Baird Publishers.

ABOUT THE AUTHOR

DR. NANCY STACKHOUSE is a university professor in elementary, early childhood, and special education in Arizona. She also works part time visiting underperforming and/or failing schools to provide findings and recommendations for improvement. Nancy earned her master's degree in special education from Arizona State University and her doctorate in curriculum and instruction from Northern Arizona University. She enjoys reading, exercising, music, concerts, meditating, traveling, and spending time with family and friends. She and her husband, Scott Stackhouse, reside in Scottsdale, Arizona.

www.ingramcontent.com/pod-product-compliance
Lightning Source LLC
Chambersburg PA
CBHW030308290526
45785CB00001B/265